Preface

The task of updating a much used and appreciated textbook is a daunting one. This is particularly so for the *Handbook of Diabetes*, which has been ubiquitous in its presence in most diabetes departments over the last decade, largely because of its clarity of text, its high quality illustrations and accessibility of information.

However, it is 6 years since the last edition and much has moved on. Moreover, previous editions have been a very recognisable offspring of the larger *Textbook of Diabetes*, which has been one of its strengths.

This edition, however, is a stand alone text that has been completely revised by the authors, independently of its larger relative but maintaining the ethos espoused in the preface to the third edition of an "easy-to-read, up-to-date and well-illustrated précis of the most important aspects of the science and clinical practice of diabetes". We have also endeavoured to make the information accessible to all professionals looking after people with diabetes. The organisation of the chapters is unchanged but their structure is broken down into sections. A list and occasional summary of landmark studies is included together with information on key websites. In addition we have included an illustrative case. Because we are increasingly working in an environment of evidence and eminence based guidelines, the text and tables include their recommendations and the source documents are listed at the end of each chapter.

References have been kept to a minimum and include as many recent reviews as possible but are inevitably a bit idiosyncratic. Apologies to those who feel we may have missed their magnum opus. Each of these features has been colour coded. A big plus is the provision of a CD of the illustrations for personal use.

The team at Wiley Blackwell have kept us to an almost impossible timetable and our thanks to Oliver Walter, Rob Blundell and Helen Harvey for their encouragement and positive feedback. Once again they have produced a beautifully laid out and illustrated text which we hope lives up to the high standards set by its predecessors.

Inevitably new information arrives while such a book is being written, so apologies if some sections seem out of date. We hope that you, the reader, will find this handbook as useful as the third edition and if so recommend it to all of your colleagues!

Rudy Bilous
Richard Donnelly

Key to the boxes

KEY POINTS

These points summarise important learning topics, things to remember and/or areas that are sometimes misunderstood by healthcare professionals.

CASE HISTORY

This is a typical case summary that illustrates a number of learning topics from the chapter.

LANDMARK CLINICAL TRIALS

These are often major trials underpinning the evidence base for clinical practice and decision-making in the area.

KEY WEBSITES

Websites that contain further information, practice guidelines and/or learning topics to supplement the information in the chapter.

FURTHER READING

Published reviews, original research or meta-analyses relevant to the chapter.

List of abbreviations

ABPI	Ankle Brachial Pressure Index		EDIC	Epidemiology of Diabetes Complications
ACE	angiotensin-converting enzyme		eGFR	estimated glomerular filtration rate
ACEI	angiotensin-converting enzyme inhibitors		EPO	erythropoietin
ADA	American Diabetes Association		ESRD	end-stage renal disease
AGE	advanced glycation endproduct		ETDRS	Early Treatment Diabetic Retinopathy Study
ALT	alanine aminotransferase			
AMI	acute myocardial infarction		FATP	fatty acid transporter protein
ARB	angiotensin type 1 receptor blocker		FDA	Food and Drug Administration
AST	aspartate aminotransferase		FFA	free fatty acids
ATP	adenosine triphosphate		FPG	fasting plasma glucose
			FSD	female sexual dysfunction
BB	BioBreeding			
BMI	Body Mass Index		GAD	glutamic acid decarboxylase
BP	blood pressure		GBM	glomerular basement membrane
			GDM	gestational diabetes mellitus
CABG	coronary artery bypass grafting		GFAT	glutamine:fructose-6-phosphate amidotransferase
CCB	calcium channel blockers			
CETP	cholesterol ester transfer protein		GFR	glomerular filtration rate
CHD	coronary heart disease		GI	gastrointestinal
CI	confidence interval		GIP	gastric inhibitory polypeptide
CIDP	chronic inflammatory demyelinating polyneuropathy		GIR	glucose infusion rate
			GLP-1	glucagon-like peptide-1
CKD	chronic kidney disease		GLUT	glucose transporter
CSF	cerebrospinal fluid			
CSII	continuous subcutaneous insulin infusion		HDL	high-density lipoprotein
CT	computed tomography		HHS	hyperosmolar hyperglycaemic state
CVD	cardiovascular disease		HL	hepatic lipase
			HLA	human leukocyte antigen
DAFNE	Dose Adjustment for Normal Eating		HOMA	Homeostasis Model Assessment
DAG	diacylglycerol		HONK	hyperosmolar non-ketotic hyperglycaemic coma
DCCT	Diabetes Control and Complications Trial			
DESMOND	Diabetes Education and Self-Management for Ongoing and Newly Diagnosed		HPLC	high-pressure liquid chromatography
			HR	hazard ratio
DKA	diabetic ketoacidosis		hsCRP	high-sensitivity C-reactive protein
DME	diabetes-related macular oedema			
DPP-4	dipeptidyl peptidase-4 (IV)		IAA	insulin autoantibody
DSN	diabetes specialist nurse		IAPP	islet amyloid polypeptide
			ICA	islet cell antibody
eAG	estimated average glucose		IDDM	insulin-dependent diabetes mellitus
ED	erectile dysfunction		IFG	impaired fasting glycaemia

IGT	impaired glucose tolerance		PAD	peripheral arterial disease
IM	intramuscular		PAI-1	plasminogen activator inhibitor-1
IPPV	intermittent positive pressure ventilation		PCI	percutaneous coronary intervention
IQR	interquartile range		PCOS	polycystic ovary syndrome
IRMA	intraretinal microvascular abnormality		PG	plasma glucose
IRS	insulin receptor substrate		PI	phospatidylinositol
ITU	intensive therapy unit		PKC	Protein kinase C
IV	intravenous		PNDM	permanent neonatal diabetes mellitus
			PP	pancreatic polypeptide
KATP	ATP-sensitive potassium channel		PPARγ	peroxisome proliferator-activated receptor-γ
			PRP	panretinal laser photocoagulation
LADA	latent autoimmune diabetes of adults			
LDL	low-density lipoprotein		QALY	quality-adjusted life-year
LH	luteinizing hormone			
			RAGE	receptor for AGE
MAP	mitogen-activated protein		RAS	renin-angiotensin system
MAPK	mitogen-activated protein kinase		RCT	randomised controlled trial
MDI	multiple daily injection		ROS	reactive oxygen species
MHC	major histocompatibility complex		RRR	relative risk reduction
MI	myocardial infarction		RRT	renal replacement therapy
MODY	maturity-onset diabetes of the young		RXR	retinoid X receptor
NADH	nicotinamide adenine dinucleotide plus hydrogen		SC	subcutaneous
			SPK	simultaneous pancreas and kidney transplantation
NADPH	nicotinamide adenine dinucleotide phosphate hydrogen		SU	sulphonylurea
NEFA	non-esterified fatty acid			
NGT	normal glucose tolerance		TCC	total contact casting
NICE	National Institute of Health and Clinical Excellence		TCF7L2	transcription factor 7-like 2 gene
			TG	triglyceride
NIDDM	non-insulin dependent diabetes mellitus		TGF	transforming growth factor
NK	natural killer		TIA	transient ischaemic attack
NKCF	natural killer cell factor		TNF	tumour necrosis factor
NLD	necrobiosis lipoidica diabeticorum		TZD	thiazolidinedione
NO	nitric oxide			
NOD	non-obese diabetic		UKPDS	UK Prospective Diabetes Study
NPH	neutral protamine Hagedorn		UTI	urinary tract infections
NPY	neuropeptide Y			
NSF	National Service Framework		VCAM	vascular cell adhesion molecule
NVD	new vessels on the disc		VDT	vibration detection threshold
NVE	new vessels elsewhere		VEGF	vascular endothelium-derived growth factor
			VIP	vasoactive intestinal peptide
OCT	optical coherence tomography		VLDL	very low-density lipoprotein
OGTT	oral glucose tolerance test			
OR	odds ratio		WHO	World Health Organization

Part 1

Introduction to diabetes

Introduction to diabetes

KEY POINTS

- Diabetes is common and its incidence is rising.
- Type 2 diabetes is by far the most common accounting for 85–95% of cases.

- Complications in the microvasculature (eye, kidney and nerve) and the macrovasculature are responsible for considerable morbidity and excess mortality.

Diabetes mellitus is a condition of chronically elevated blood glucose concentrations which give rise to its main symptom of passing large quantities of sweet-tasting urine (*diabetes* from the Greek word meaning 'a siphon', as the body acts as a conduit for the excess fluid, and *mellitus* from the Greek and Latin for honey). The fundamental underlying abnormality is a net (relative or absent) deficiency of the hormone insulin. Insulin is essentially the only hormone that can lower blood glucose.

There are two categories of diabetes: type 1 is caused by an autoimmune destruction of the insulin-producing β cell of the islets of Langerhans in the pancreas (absolute deficiency); and type 2 is a result of both impaired insulin secretion and resistance to its action – often secondary to obesity (relative deficiency).

The precise level of blood glucose that defines diabetes has been revised several times and is covered in more detail in Chapter 3. Diabetes is common and is becoming more common. Age-adjusted prevalence is set to rise from 5.9% to 7.1% (246–380 million) worldwide in the 20–79 year age group, a 55% increase (Figure 1.1). The relative proportions of type 1 to type 2 vary from 15:85 for Western populations to 5:95 in developing countries.

Handbook of Diabetes, 4th edition. By © Rudy Bilous & Richard Donnelly. Published 2010 by Blackwell Publishing Ltd.

It is the short- and long-term complications of diabetes which make it a major public health problem. Absolute deficiency of insulin leads to ketoacidosis and coma with an appreciable mortality even in the UK and other Western countries. Hyperglycaemic hyperosmolar coma (now called hyperglycaemic hyperosmolar state) is less common and more insidious but remains an equally serious problem for people with type 2 diabetes (see Chapter 12).

Long-term hyperglycaemia affects the microvasculature of the eye, kidney and nerve as well as the larger arteries, leading to accelerated atherosclerosis. Diabetes is the most common cause of blindness in those of working age, the most common single cause of end-stage renal failure worldwide, and the consequences of neuropathy make it the most common cause of non-traumatic lower limb amputation. Mortality from ischaemic heart disease and stroke is 2–4-fold higher than in the age- and sex-matched non-diabetic population. All these important clinical problems will be covered in detail in subsequent chapters (Figure 1.2).

This handbook sets out to cover the essentials of diagnosis, epidemiology and management of diabetes and its distressingly many complications. By using case vignettes and summaries of key trials together with web links and suggestions for further reading, it will serve as a useful desktop reference for all healthcare professionals who provide diabetes care.

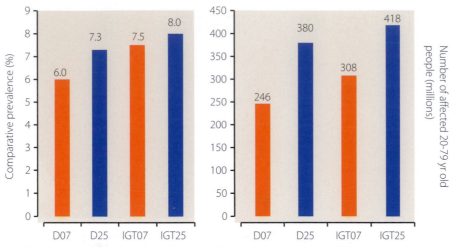

Figure 1.1 Estimated comparative prevalence (age adjusted) of diabetes and impaired glucose tolerance (IGT) together with numbers affected for the global population age 20–79 years for 2007 (red) and 2025 (blue). Data from *Diabetes Atlas*, 3rd edn, International Diabetes Federation.

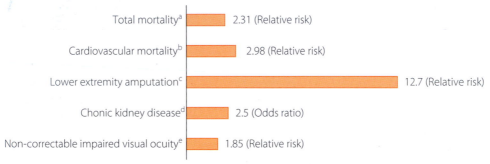

Figure 1.2 Rates of major complications of diabetes for the US population derived from NHANES or Medicare data. [a]NHANES data 1988–2000; [b]Medicare population Minnesota 1993–5; [c]NHANES data, 1999–2006 (chronic kidney disease defined as estimated GFR <60 mL/min/1.73 m^2.); [d]NHANES data, 1999–2002.

FURTHER READING

International Diabetes Federation. *Diabetes Atlas*, 4th edn. Brussels: International Diabetes Federation, 2009.

KEY WEBSITE

- Diabetes Atlas: www.eatlas.idf.org

Chapter 2

History of diabetes

KEY POINTS

- Diabetes has been known since ancient times.
- A link to the pancreas was established in 1889 culminating in the isolation of insulin in 1921.
- The structure of insulin was finally elucidated in the 1960s.
- Insulin was the first therapy to be manufactured using genetic engineering techniques.

Diseases with the clinical features of diabetes have been recognised since antiquity. The Ebers papyrus (Figure 2.1), dating from 1550 BC, describes a polyuric state that resembles diabetes.

The word 'diabetes' was first used by Aretaeus of Cappadocia in the second century AD. Aretaeus gave a clinical description of the disease (Box 2.1), noting the increased urine flow, thirst and weight loss, features that are instantly recognizable today.

The sweet, honey-like taste of urine in polyuric states, which attracted ants and other insects, was reported by Hindu physicians such as Sushrut (Susruta) during the fifth and sixth centuries AD. These descriptions even mention two forms of diabetes, the more common occurring in older, overweight and indolent people, and the other in lean people who did not survive for long. This empirical subdivision predicted the modern classification into type 1 and type 2 diabetes.

Diabetes was largely neglected in Europe until a 17th-century English physician, Thomas Willis (1621–75) (Figure 2.2), rediscovered the sweetness of diabetic urine. Willis, who was physician to King Charles II, thought that the disease had been rare in ancient times, but that its frequency was increasing in his age 'given to good fellowship'. Nearly a century later, the Liverpool physician Matthew Dobson (1735–84) showed that the sweetness of urine and serum was caused by sugar. John Rollo (d. 1809) was the first to apply the adjective 'mellitus' to the disease.

In the 19th century, the French physiologist Claude Bernard (1813–78) (Figure 2.3) made many discoveries relating to diabetes. Among these was the finding that the sugar that appears in the urine was stored in the liver as glycogen. Bernard also demonstrated links between the central nervous system and diabetes when he observed

Handbook of Diabetes, 4th edition. By © Rudy Bilous & Richard Donnelly. Published 2010 by Blackwell Publishing Ltd.

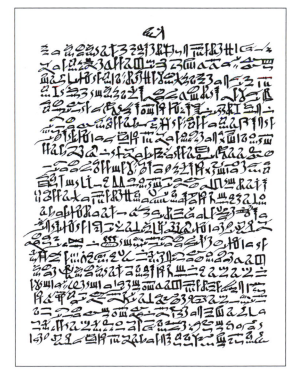

Figure 2.1 The Ebers papyrus. The Wellcome Institute Library, London, UK.

Box 2.1 Description of diabetes by Aretaeus

Diabetes is a dreadful affliction, not very frequent among men, being a melting down of the flesh and limbs into urine. The patients never stop making water and the flow is incessant, like the opening of aqueducts. Life is short, unpleasant and painful, thirst unquenchable, drinking excessive, and disproportionate to the large quantity of urine, for yet more urine is passed. One cannot stop them either from drinking or making water. If for a while they abstain from drinking, their mouths become parched and their bodies dry; the viscera seem scorched up, the patients are affected by nausea, restlessness and a burning thirst, and within a short time, they expire.

Adapted from Papaspyros S. *The History of Diabetes Mellitus*, 2nd edn. Stuttgart: Thieme, 1964.

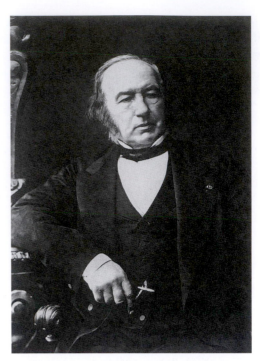

Figure 2.3 Claude Bernard. The Wellcome Institue Library, London, UK.

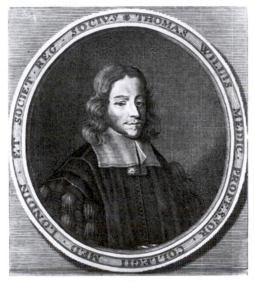

Figure 2.2 Thomas Willis. The Wellcome Institue Library, London, UK.

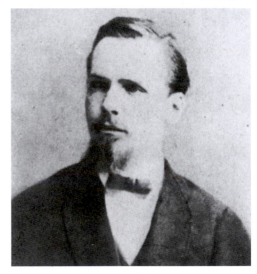

Figure 2.4 Paul Langerhans. The Wellcome Institue Library, London, UK.

temporary hyperglycaemia (piqûre diabetes) when the medulla of conscious rabbits was transfixed with a needle.

In 1889, Oskar Minkowski (1858–1931) and Joseph von Mering (1849–1908) from Strasbourg removed the pancreas from a dog to see if the organ was essential for life. The animal displayed typical signs of diabetes, with thirst, polyuria and wasting, which were associated with glycosuria and hyperglycaemia. This experiment showed that a pancreatic disorder causes diabetes, but they did not follow up on the observation.

Paul Langerhans (1847–88) (Figure 2.4) from Berlin, in his doctoral thesis of 1869, was the first to describe small clusters of cells in teased preparations of the pancreas. He did not speculate on the function of the cells, and it was Edouard Laguesse in France who later (1893) named the cells 'islets of Langerhans' and suggested that they were endocrine tissue of the pancreas that produced a glucose-lowering hormone.

In the early 20th century, several workers isolated impure hypoglycaemic extracts from the pancreas, including the Berlin physician Georg Zuelzer (1840–1949), the Romanian Nicolas Paulesco (1869–1931), and the Americans Ernest Scott (1877–1966) and Israel Kleiner (1885–1966).

Insulin was discovered in 1921 at the University of Toronto, Canada, through a collaboration between the surgeon Frederick G Banting (1891–1941), his student assistant Charles H Best (1899–1978), the biochemist James B Collip (1892–1965) and the physiologist JJR Macleod (1876–1935). Banting and Best made chilled extracts of dog pancreas, injected them into pancreatectomised diabetic dogs, and showed a fall in blood gluocse concentrations (Figure 2.5).

Banting and Best's notes of the dog experiments refer to the administration of 'isletin', later called insulin by them at the suggestion of Macleod. They were unaware that the Belgian Jean de Meyer had already coined the term 'insuline' in 1909. (All these names ultimately derive from the Latin for 'island'.)

Collip improved the methods for the extraction and purification of insulin from the pancreas, and the first diabetic patient, a 14-year-old boy called Leonard Thompson, was treated on 11th January 1922. A commercially viable extraction procedure was then developed in collaboration with chemists from Eli Lilly and Co. in the USA, and insulin became widely available in North America and Europe from 1923. The 1923 Nobel Prize for Physiology or Medicine was awarded to Banting and Macleod, who decided to share their prizes with Best and Collip.

The American physician Elliot P Joslin (1869–1962) was one of the first doctors to gain experience with insulin. Working in Boston, he treated 293 patients in the first year after August 1922. Joslin also introduced systematic education for his diabetic patients.

In the UK, the discovery of insulin saved the life of the London physician Robin D Lawrence (1892–1968), who had recently developed type 1 diabetes. He subsequently played a leading part in the founding of the British Diabetic Association (now Diabetes UK).

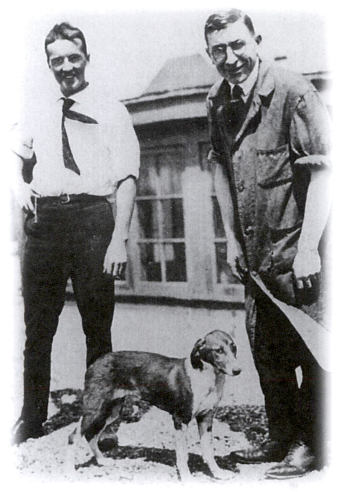

Figure 2.5 Charles Best and Frederick Banting in Toronto in 1922 (the dog is thought to have been called Marjorie).

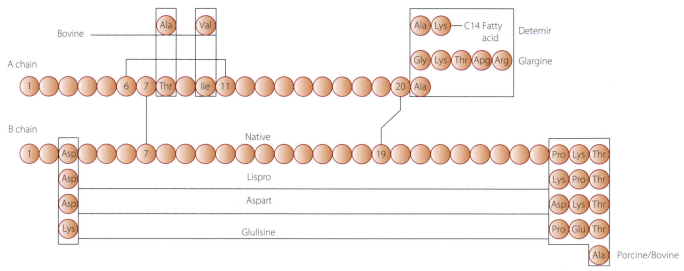

Figure 2.6 Schematic amino acid sequence of human insulin; porcine and bovine insulin; the short-acting insulin analogues aspart, lispro and glulisine; and the long-acting analogues glargine and detemir.

Among the many major advances since the introduction of insulin into clinical practice was the elucidation in 1955 of its primary structure (amino acid sequence) (Figure 2.6) by the Cambridge UK scientist Frederick Sanger (b. 1918), who received the Nobel Prize for this work in 1958.

Oxford-based Dorothy Hodgkin (1910–1994), another Nobel Prize winner, and her colleagues described the three-dimensional structure of insulin using X-ray crystallography (1969).

By the 1950s, it was accepted that tissue complications, such as those that occur in the eye and kidney, continued to develop in long-standing diabetes, in spite of insulin treatment. The definitive proof that normalization of glycaemia could prevent or delay the development of diabetic complications had to wait until 1993 for type 1 diabetes (the Diabetes Control and Complications Trial in North America) and 1998 for type 2 diabetes (the UK Prospective Diabetes Study – UKPDS).

Until the 1980s, insulin was derived only from animal pancreata, in increasingly more refined preparations. Using additives such as protamine or zinc, the subcutaneous absorption could be delayed, thus providing 24-hour availability using 2–4 injections a day of different preparations.

With the development of genetic engineering, it became possible to produce human insulin and subsequent further manipulations of the molecule have led to a wide range of preparations with different absorption profiles (Figure 2.6). Further developments along these lines are expected but a continuing dependence upon subcutaneous injection as the main route of administration is likely for the foreseeable future.

In type 2 diabetes oral agents have been available since the 1950s. It is now possible, however, to modify both insulin secretion and its action by using drugs that both increase insulin release from the β cell and improve insulin sensitivity peripherally. There is intensive research into therapies for diabetes and newer agents will undoubtedly become available as our understanding of the mechanism of glucose homeostasis increases.

These therapeutic areas will be covered in more detail in subsequent chapters.

FURTHER READING

Bliss M. *The Discovery of Insulin*. Toronto: McLelland and Stewart, 1982.

Diagnosis and classification of diabetes

Diabetes mellitus is diagnosed by identifying chronic hyperglycaemia. The World Health Organization (WHO) and the American Diabetes Association (ADA) have used a fasting plasma glucose (FPG) of 7 mmol/L or higher to define diabetes (Table 3.1). This originated from epidemiological studies in the 1990s which appeared to show that the risk of microvascular complications (e.g. retinopathy) increases sharply at a FPG threshold of 7 mmol/L (Figure 3.1). Lately, however, the notion of a clear glycaemic threshold separating people at high and low risk of diabetic microvascular complications has been called into question. Part of the rationale for switching to $HbA_{1c} > 6.5\%$ (48 mmol/mol) as a diagnostic test is that moderate retinopathy, in more recent trials, is rare below this HbA_{1c} threshold.

There are currently 23.6 million people in the USA with diabetes (7.8% of the population). The total number of people with diabetes worldwide is projected to increase from 171 million in 2000 to 366 million in 2030. A key demographic change to the rising prevalence of diabetes worldwide is an increasing proportion of people >65 years of age.

Table 3.1 Classification of diabetes and glucose intolerance according to ADA fasting and WHO 2-h glucose criteria. To convert glucose concentrations from mmol/L into mg/dL, multiply by 18

	Blood sample		
	Plasma	**Capillary**	**Whole**
Fasting blood glucose (mmol/L)			
Normal	<6.1	<5.6	<5.6
Impaired fasting glycaemia	6.1–6.9	5.6–6.0	5.6–6.0
Diabetes	≥7.0	≥6.1	≥6.1
2-hour blood glucose			
Normal	<7.8	<7.8	<6.7
Impaired glucose tolerance	7.8–11.0	7.8–11.0	6.7–9.9
Diabetes	≥11.1	≥11.1	≥10.0

Diabetes can be diagnosed in several ways.
- $HbA_{1c} \geq 6.5\%$ (48 mmol/mol).
- A casual (random) plasma glucose level ≥11.1 mmol/L (200 mg/dL) in someone with typical symptoms of diabetes.
- A fasting plasma glucose level ≥7.0 mmol/L (126 mg/dL).
- A plasma glucose level ≥11.1 mmol/L (200 mg/dL) 2 hours after a 75 g load of glucose given by mouth (the oral glucose tolerance test – OGTT).

Handbook of Diabetes, 4th edition. By © Rudy Bilous & Richard Donnelly. Published 2010 by Blackwell Publishing Ltd.

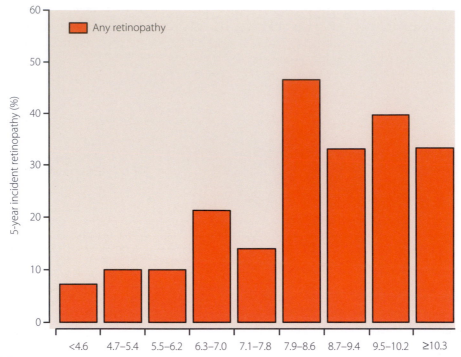

Figure 3.1 Relationship between FPG and incident retinopathy in the Blue Moutains Eye study. In more recent studies (using better methods for detecting retinopathy) there is no evidence of a threshold effect at 7 mmol/L. The risk of retinopathy is continuous. It is reassuring that significant retinopathy is extremely rare in individuals with HbA$_{1c}$ below the diagnosis threshold of 6.5% (48 mmol/mol). Adapted from Wong et al. Lancet 2008; 371: 736–743.

Box 3.1 Some features of impaired glucose tolerance and/or impaired fasting glycaemia

- Intermediate stage of disordered glucose metabolism
- Increased risk of progression to diabetes
- Increased risk of cardiovascular disease
- Little or no risk of microvascular disease
- Some patients may revert to normoglycaemiaic
- IFG is predictive of future type 2 diabetes, whereas IGT is more predictive of CV risk

LANDMARK CLINICAL TRIALS

DECODE Study Group. Glucose tolerance and mortality: comparison of WHO and American Diabetes Association diagnostic criteria. Lancet 1999; 354: 617–621.

Diabetes Prevention Program Research Group. The prevalence of retinopathy in impaired glucose tolerance and recent-onset diabetes in the Diabetes Prevention Program. Diabetic Med 2007; 24: 137–144.

Harjutsalo V, Sjoberg L, Tuomilehto J. Time trends in the incidence of type 1 diabetes in Finnish children. Lancet 2008; 371: 1777–1782.

Li G, Zhang P, Wang J, et al. The long-term effect of lifestyle interventions to prevent diabetes in the China Da Qing Diabetes Prevention Study: a 20-year follow-up study. Lancet 2008; 371: 1783–1789.

Tabak AG, Jokela M, Akbaraly T, et al. Trajectories of glycaemia, insulin sensitivity, and insulin secretion before diagnosis of type 2 diabetes: an analysis from the Whitehall II study. Lancet 2009; 373: 2215–2221.

Wild S, Roglic G, Green A, et al. Global prevalence of diabetes: estimates for the year 2000 and projections for 2030. Diabetes Care 2004; 27: 1047–1053.

Wong TY, Liew G, Tapp R, et al. Relation between fasting glucose and retinopathy for diagnosis of diabetes: three population-based cross-sectional studies. Lancet 2008; 371: 736–743.

Intermediate categories of hyperglycaemia: prediabetes

During the natural history of all forms of diabetes, the disease passes through a stage of impaired glucose tolerance (IGT), defined as a plasma glucose of 7.8–11.0 mmol/L (140–200 mg/dL) 2 hours after an OGTT. Impaired fasting glycaemia (IFG) is an analogous category based on fasting glucose levels, and is defined as a FPG of 6.1–6.9 mmol/L (110–126 mg/dL) (Box 3.1).

Impaired glucose tolerance and IFG are intermediate metabolic stages between normal glucose homeostasis and diabetes. They are both risk factors for future diabetes and cardiovascular disease, but the 2-hour plasma glucose concentration is a particularly strong predictor of cardiovascular risk and mortality (Figure 3.2).

A proportion of patients with IFG and/or IGT (5–10% per annum) will deteriorate metabolically into overt diabetes. Lifestyle modification (diet, exercise and weight loss) is the best approach to diabetes prevention for these patients. More recently, some genetic markers have been associated with an increased risk of progression from IGT to diabetes, e.g. common polymorphisms of the transcription factor 7-like 2 gene (TCF7L2).

For an OGTT, the subject is tested in the morning after an overnight fast, in the seated position. After taking a fasting blood sample, 75 g of glucose is given by mouth, often in the form of a glucose drink such as Lucozade (388 mL). For children, the glucose dose is calculated as 1.75 g/kg. A further blood sample is taken at 2 hours, and the fasting and 2-hour glucose values are interpreted as in Figure 3.3.

Screening for diabetes by the FPG level does not identify exactly the same population as that diagnosed by the plasma glucose 2 hours after an OGTT or by HbA_{1c} (Table 3.2). For example, in the US NHANES study, 1.6% of the population had HbA_{1c} ≥6.5% but 5% of these would be undiagnosed using FPG or 2h criteria. Only 55% of patients with FPG ≥ 7mmol/L and 2h glucose ≥11.1 mmol/L had an HbA_{1c} ≥6.5% (Cowie et al. 2010).

Glycosuria (the presence of glucose in the urine) cannot be used to diagnose diabetes because of the poor relationship between blood and urine glucose. This is for several reasons: the renal threshold for glucose reabsorption varies considerably within and between individuals, the urine glucose concentration is affected by the subject's state of

Table 3.2 Use of HbA_{1c} ≥ 6.5% (48 mmol/mol) as a cut-off for making the diagnosis of diabetes offers some advantages but there are several potential disadvantages

Advantages	Disadvantages

• Avoids the need for a fasting blood sample, and the pre-analytical instability of glucose measurements
• HbA_{1c} reflects glycaemia over several weeks
• Lower biological variability of HbA_{1c} compared with FPG or 2h glucose
• Virtual absence of significant retinopathy among people with HbA_{1c} < 6.5%
	• HbA_{1c} measurements can give spurious results in:
	  ○ anaemia (Fe-deficiency)
	  ○ haemoglobinopathies
	  ○ renal failure
	  ○ different ethnic groups
	• Diagnosis by HbA_{1c} will identify a different population to that diagnosed by FPG
	• Distribution of HbA_{1c} values varies in different ethnic groups
	• HbA_{1c} increases with age
	• Some patients and ethnic groups may be diagnosed with diabetes by some criteria but not others

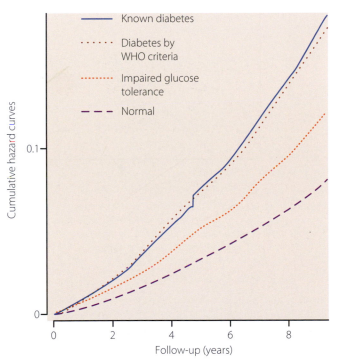

Figure 3.2 The relationship between 2-hour plasma glucose and survival in patients with normal glucose tolerance, patients with IGT, those with newly diagnosed diabetes by OGTT, and those with known diabetes, as shown by the DECODE study (combining data from 13 European cohort studies). Reproduced from DECODE Study Group. Lancet 1999; 354: 617–621.

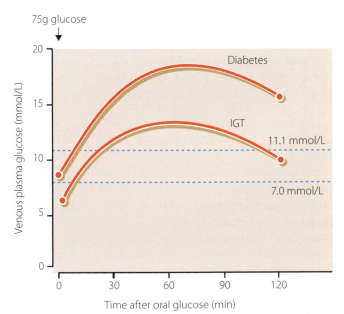

Figure 3.3 Diagnosis of diabetes and IGT by the oral glucose tolerance test.

Table 3.3 Historically, HbA$_{1c}$ has been reported in percentage values describing the proportion of haemoglobin that is glycated. The assay was aligned to that used in the Diabetes Control and Complications (DCCT) trial. The International Federation of Clinical Chemistry (IFCC) has now established a new reference system, and values will be reported in mmol HbA$_{1c}$ per mol haemoglobin without glucose attached. Conversion for HbA$_{1c}$ is shown below

DCCT (%)	IFCC (mmol/mol)	DCCT (%)	IFCC (mmol/mol)
6.0	42	9.0	75
6.2	44	9.2	77
6.4	46	9.4	79
6.5	48	9.5	80
6.6	49	9.6	81
6.8	51	9.8	84
7.0	53	10.0	86
7.2	55	10.2	88
7.4	57	10.4	90
7.5	58	10.5	91
7.6	60	10.6	92
7.8	62	10.8	95
8.0	64	11.0	97
8.2	66	11.2	99
8.4	68	11.4	101
8.5	69	11.5	102
8.6	70	11.6	103
8.8	73	11.8	105

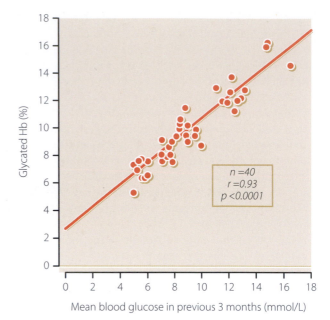

Figure 3.4 HbA$_{1c}$ correlates well with previous mean blood glucose levels over several weeks. From Paisey. Diabetologia 1980; 19: 31–34.

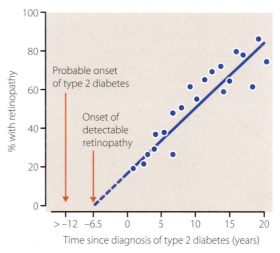

Figure 3.5 The prevalence of retinopathy in type 2 diabetes relative to the time of clinical diagnosis. Note the presence of retinopathy at diagnosis and the likely onset of retinopathy and diabetes some years before diagnosis. From Harris et al. Diabetes Care 1992; 15: 815–819.

hydration and the result reflects the average blood glucose during the period that urine has accumulated in the bladder. The average renal threshold is 10 mmol/L (i.e. blood glucose concentration above this level will 'spill over' into the urine), but a negative urine test can be associated with marked hyperglycaemia.

Longer term indices of hyperglycaemia include the glycated haemoglobin percentage (HbA$_{1c}$), a measure of integrated blood glucose control over the preceding few weeks. HbA$_{1c}$ is used primarily to assess glycaemic control among people with diabetes on treatment (aiming for HbA$_{1c}$ 6–7%). HbA$_{1c}$ analyses are now being calibrated to the IFCC assay(rather than the NGSP DCCT HPLC assay). Thus, the units of HbA$_{1c}$ are changing from percent to mmol/mol (Table 3.3).

The potential value of screening for diabetes is to facilitate early diagnosis and treatment. About 20% of newly diagnosed subjects with types 2 diabetes already have evidence of vascular complications. This suggests that complications begin about 5–6 years before a diagnosis is made, and that the actual onset of (type 2) diabetes may occur several years before the clinical diagnosis.

In most countries, there is no systematic screening policy for diabetes, yet there are estimates that up to 50% of patients with diabetes are undiagnosed. *Ad hoc* screening of high-risk groups is becoming more common. The FPG is quick and cheap, but can miss those with isolated postchallenge hyperglycaemia. In future, HbA$_{1c}$ will be increasingly used for screening and diagnosis. Screening policies should target high-risk groups (Box 3.2).

Classification of diabetes

The current classification of diabetes is based on the aetiology of the disease (Box 3.3). There are four categories.

Box 3.2 High-risk patients who should be screened annually for type 2 diabetes

- Metabolic syndrome
- Patients >45 years of age, especially the obese
- Those with parents or siblings with type 2 diabetes
- Ethnic minorities, e.g. South Indians, even if non-obese
- Patients with cardiovascular risk factors, e.g. hypertension or dyslipidaemia, and those with established atherosclerotic disease
- Women with previous gestational diabetes
- Women with polycystic ovary syndrome
- Patients with IFG/IGT

Box 3.3 Classification of diabetes

- Type 1 (β cell destruction, usually leading to absolute insulin deficiency)
  - Autoimmune
  - Idiopathic
- Type 2
  - Ranges from predominantly insulin resistant, with relative insulin deficiency, to a predominantly insulin-secretory defect, with or without insulin resistance
- Other specific types
  - Genetic defects of β cell function
  - Genetic defects of insulin action
  - Diseases of exocrine pancreas
  - Endocrinopathies
  - Drug induced or chemical induced, e.g. steroids
  - Infections
  - Uncommon forms of immune-mediated diabetes
  - Other genetic syndromes sometimes associated with diabetes
- Gestational diabetes

CASE HISTORY

A 66-year-old retired policeman attends his family doctor for a routine blood pressure (BP) check. He has had hypertension for 4 years. He reports incidentally that he has been feeling generally tired and lethargic. On further questioning, he admits to nocturia ×3 and volunteers that in recent months he has been taking a glass of water to bed since he often wakes feeling thirsty. The GP notices that he had a cutaneous boil lanced 6 weeks ago. Apart from hypertension, there is no other significant past medical history but his bodyweight has gradually risen (95 kg, Body Mass Index (BMI) 32). He takes an angiotensin-converting enzyme (ACE) inhibitor, lisinopril 10 mg, for hypertension. His mother had type 2 diabetes, he is a non-smoker and drinks 15 units of alcohol per week. His only exercise is golf, twice per week. The doctor takes a random venous blood sample, which shows a plasma glucose level of 13 mmol/L. Further blood tests show a normal haematology profile, normal electrolytes and renal function, HbA_{1c} 8.3%, and fasting lipids show total cholesterol 6.6 mmol/L, low-density lipoprotein (LDL)-cholesterol 4.3 mmol/L, triglycerides 3.9 mmol/L and high-density lipoprotein (HDL)-cholesterol 0.6 mmol/L. Minor abnormalities of liver function are also noted (aspartate aminotransferase (AST) and alanine aminotransferase (ALT) 2–3× upper limit).

Comment: This man presents with typical symptoms of type 2 diabetes and several risk factors (age, obesity, hypertension, family history). The random plasma glucose, in the context of symptoms, is diagnostic. He has features of the metabolic syndrome, including hypertension, dyslipidaemia (high triglycerides and low HDL-cholesterol) and central obesity, and fatty infiltration of the liver is common in this scenario. The HbA_{1c} is quite high, reflecting chronic hyperglycaemia over at least 8 weeks. Susceptibility to infections is typical.

- Type 1 diabetes (caused by pancreatic islet cell destruction).
- Type 2 diabetes (caused by a combination of insulin resistance and β cell insulin secretory dysfunction).
- Other specific types of diabetes (caused by conditions such as endocrinopathies, diseases of the exocrine pancreas, genetic syndromes, etc.; see below).
- Gestational diabetes (defined as diabetes that occurs for the first time in pregnancy).

Type 1 diabetes is subdivided into two main types: 1a or autoimmune (about 90% of type 1 patients in Europe and North America, in which immune markers, such as circulating islet cell antibodies, suggest autoimmune destruction of the β cells) and 1b or idiopathic (where there is no evidence of autoimmunity).

A steady increase (2.5–3% per annum) in the incidence of type 1 diabetes has been reported worldwide, especially among young children <4 years old. There are large differences between countries in the incidence of type 1 diabetes, e.g. up to 10-fold difference among European countries.

This classification has now replaced the earlier, clinical classification into 'insulin-dependent diabetes mellitus' (IDDM) and 'non-insulin dependent diabetes mellitus' (NIDDM), which was based on the need for insulin treatment at diagnosis. IDDM is broadly equivalent to type 1 diabetes and NIDDM to type 2 diabetes (Table 3.4). One of the disadvantages of the old classification according to treatment was that subjects could change their type of diabetes – for example, some type 1a patients diagnosed after the age of 40 years masquerade as NIDDM, before eventually becoming truly insulin dependent (this is now classified as latent autoimmune diabetes in adults; LADA).

Table 3.4 Type 1 and 2 diabetes correspond to IDDM and NIDDM in the old classification system

IDDM	NIDDM
Type 1	Type 2
LADA (late stage)	LADA (early stage)

Various clinical and biochemical features can be used to decide whether the patient has type 1 or type 2 diabetes (Box 3.4). The distinction may be difficult in individual cases.

The category of 'other specific types of diabetes' is a large group of conditions (Box 3.5), which includes genetic defects in insulin secretion (such as in maturity-onset diabetes of the young (MODY) and insulinopathies), genetic defects in insulin action (e.g. syndromes of severe insulin resistance), pancreatitis and other exocrine disorders, hormone-secreting tumours such as acromegaly (growth hormone)

Box 3.4 Clinical features of type 1 and type 2 diabetes

Type 1 diabetes
- Sudden onset with severe symptoms of thirst and ketoacidosis (vomiting, hyperventilation, dehydration)
- Recent, marked weight loss. Usually lean
- Spontaneous ketosis
- Life-threatening; needs urgent insulin replacement
- Absent C-peptide
- Markers of autoimmunity present (e.g. islet cell antibodies)

Type 2 diabetes
- Usually insidious onset of tiredness, thirst, polyuria, nocturia
- No ketoacidosis
- Usually overweight or obese; often no recent weight loss
- Frequent infections, e.g. urine, skin, chest
- Symptoms may be minimal and/or ignored by patient
- Often other features of 'metabolic syndrome', e.g. hypertension
- C-peptide detectable

Box 3.5 Other specific types of diabetes

Genetic defects of β cell function
- Chromosome 12, HNF-1a (formerly MODY-3)
- Chromosome 7, glucokinase (formerly MODY-2)
- Chromosome 20, HNF-4a (formerly MODY-1)
- Mitochondrial DNA
- Insulinopathies

Genetic defects in insulin action
- Type A insulin resistance
- Leprechaunism
- Rabson–Mendenhall syndrome
- Lipoatrophic diabetes

Diseases of the exocrine pancreas
- Pancreatitis
- Trauma/pancreatectomy
- Neoplasia
- Cystic fibrosis
- Haemochromatosis
- Fibrocalculous pancreatopathy

Endocrinopathies
- Acromegaly
- Cushing's syndrome
- Glucagonoma
- Phaeochromocytoma
- Hyperthyroidism
- Somatostatinoma
- Aldosteronoma

Drug induced or chemical induced
- Glucocorticoids
- Thiazides
- Pentamidine
- Nicotinic acid
- Thyroid hormone
- β-adrenergic agonists
- Interferon-α

Infections
- Congenital rubella
- Cytomegalovirus
- Others
- Uncommon forms of immune-mediated diabetes
- 'Stiff man' syndrome
- Anti-insulin receptor antibodies

Other genetic syndromes sometimes associated with diabetes
- Down's syndrome
- Klinefelter's syndrome
- Turner's syndrome
- Wolfram's syndrome
- Friedreich's ataxia
- Huntington's chorea
- Lawrence–Moon–Biedl syndrome
- Myotonic dystrophy
- Porphyria
- Prader–Willi syndrome

and Cushing's syndrome (cortisol). Some cases are cau
by the administration of drugs such as glucocorticoids. Some
genetic syndromes are sometimes associated with diabetes
(e.g. Down's syndrome, Klinefelter's syndrome and many
more).

FURTHER READING

American Diabetes Association. Diagnosis and classification of diabetes mellitus. Diabetes Care 2010; 33(Suppl 1): S62–S69.

Arky RA. 'Doctor, is my sugar normal?' N Engl J Med 2005; 353: 1511–1513.

Avenell A, Broom J, Brown TJ, et al. Screening for type 2 diabetes: literature review and economic modelling. Health Technol Assess 2007; 11: 1–125.

Bloomgarden Z. A1c: Recommendations, debates and questions. Diabetes Care 2009; 32: e141–e147.

Cowie CC, Rust KF, Boyd-Holt DD, et al. Prevalence of diabetes and high risk for diabetes using A1c criteria in the US population in 1988–2006. Diabetes Care 2010; 33: 562–568.

Christensen DL, Witte DR, Kaduka L, et al. Moving to an A1c-based diagnosis of diabetes has a different impact on prevalence in different ethnic groups. Diabetes Care 2010; 33: 580–582.

Eddy DM, Schlessinger L, Kahn R. Clinical outcomes and cost-effectiveness of strategies for managing people at high risk for diabetes. Ann Intern Med 2005; 143: 251–264.

Florez JC, Jablonski K, Bayley N, et al. TCF7L2 polymorphisms and progression to diabetes in the Diabetes Prevention Program. N Engl J Med 2006; 355: 241–250.

Gillies CL, Lambert P, Abrams K, et al. Different strategies for screening and prevention of type 2 diabetes in adults: cost effectiveness analysis. BMJ 2008; 336: 1180–1184.

Glumer C, Yuyun M, Griffin S, et al. What determines the cost-effectiveness of diabetes screening? Diabetologia 2006; 49: 1536–1544.

Harris MI, Klein R, Welborn T, et al. Onset of NIDDM occurs at least 4–7 years before clinical diagnosis. Diabet Care 1992; 15: 815–819.

International Expert Committee Report (ADA-EASD-IDF) on the role of the A1c assay in the diagnosis of diabetes. Diabetes Care 2009; 32: 1327–1334.

Public health aspects of diabetes

Impact on healthcare expenditure

Diabetes is an expensive disease. About 75% of the direct costs are absorbed by the long-term complications, rather than the management of diabetes itself. In the USA in 2002, the annual economic burden of diabetes was estimated at $132 billion (accounting for >10% of total US healthcare expenditure). About 75% of the direct costs are attributable to managing the longterm vascular complications of diabetes, and 90% of resources are spent on type 2 diabetes. In terms of the costs of managing hyperglycaemia, self-monitoring of blood glucose concentrations is the single biggest item.

The management of diabetes is becoming more complex and more intensive, and therefore more expensive (Figure 4.1). The mean number of diabetes medications per treated patient increased from 1.14 in 1994 to 1.63 in 2007. Recent trends in the use of newer insulins and oral antidiabetic drugs have resulted in extra costs (mean cost per prescription in the USA increased from $56 in 2001 to $76 in 2007). Overall, drug expenditure in the US rose from $6.7 billion in 2001 to $12.5 billion in 2007.

There is an increasing awareness of the clinical and cost-effectiveness of diabetes interventions on the longer term outcomes. Based on the UK Prospective Diabetes Study (UKPDS), each quality-adjusted life-year (QALY) gained by intensive blood glucose control cost approximately £6028 (in 2004 values). In contrast, the equivalent cost for implementing an intensive blood pressure (BP) control policy was only £369. Both of these estimates are well below the threshold, or affordability index, of £20,000 per QALY set by the UK National Institute of Health and Clinical Excellence (NICE) when advising on the use of a new technology in the National Health Service (NHS). In particular, the total annual cost of providing UKPDS treatment to reduce diabetes complications amounted to <1% of the UK NHS budget for 2001–5.

Health economic analyses in the US have shown that a 50-year-old patient recently diagnosed with diabetes has an annual medical expenditure that is $4174 greater than an identical person without diabetes. Furthermore, each additional year with diabetes increases the annual medical expenditure by $158 over and above the increases in medical costs attributable to ageing (Figure 4.2).

Patterns of survival and cardiovascular outcomes

The overall life expectancy of patients with diabetes is reduced by about 25%, and cardiovascular disease accounts for three-quarters of all deaths among patients with diabetes.

Handbook of Diabetes, 4th edition. By © Rudy Bilous & Richard Donnelly. Published 2010 by Blackwell Publishing Ltd.

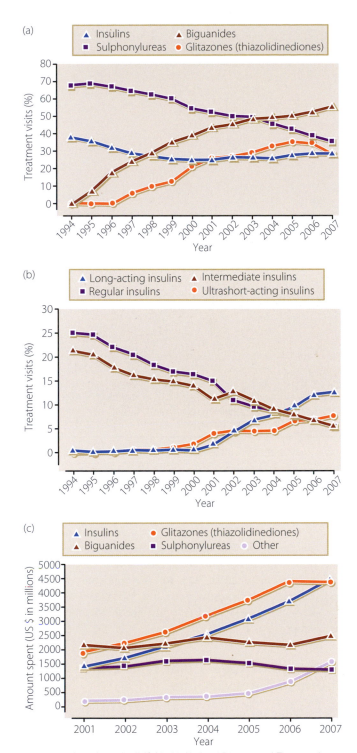

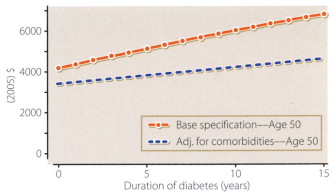

Figure 4.2 This graph shows the average incremental cost of diabetes as a function of the number of years with diabetes. Under the base specification, a 50-year-old person just diagnosed with diabetes has medical expenditures that are $4174 higher than an identical person without diabetes. A 50-year-old patient who has had diabetes for 10 years has medical expenditures that are $6054 greater than an identical person without diabetes (2005 values). Adapted from Trogdon & Hylands. *Diabetes Care* 2008; 31: 2307–2311.

Table 4.1 Causes of death in patients with type 1 and type 2 diabetes. From Marks HH, Krall LP. In: Marble A et al. (eds) *Joslin's Diabetes Mellitus*, 12th edn. Philadelphia: Lea and Febiger, 1988: 209–254

	Type 1 (%)	Type 2 (%)
Cardiovascular disease	15	58
Cerebrovascular disease	3	12
Nephropathy	55	3
Diabetic coma	4	1
Malignancy	0	11
Infections	10	4
Others	13	11

Figure 4.1 Data from the IMS Health National Disease and Therapeutic Index (USA) showing national trends in America over recent years: (a) trends in the use of insulins, sulphonylureas, biguanides and glitazones from 1994 to 2007; (b) the use of different types of insulin (1994–2007); and (c) the amount spent per year on diabetes drugs (2001–2007); 'other' includes insulin secretagogues (e.g. nateglinide), α-glucosidase inhibitors (e.g. acarbose), DPP-4 inhibitors (e.g. sitagliptin) and GLP-1 agonists (e.g. exenatide). Adapted from Alexander et al. *Arch Intern Med* 2008; 168: 2088–2094.

Diabetes confers an equivalent risk to ageing 15 years. The causes of death are proportionately different in type 1 and type 2 diabetes (Table 4.1). In long-duration type 1 diabetes, for example, nephropathy and heart disease are common, whereas in type 2 diabetes most deaths are due to premature cardiovascular disease (coronary heart disease and stroke). After adjustment for other risk factors, an increase in HbA$_{1c}$ of 1% is associated with an 18% increase in the risk of a cardiovascular event and a 12–14% increase in the risk of death.

Type 1 diabetes is associated with at least a 10-fold increase in cardiovascular disease compared with an age-matched population without diabetes, and in recent years mortality rates from type 1 diabetes have been falling in many countries as a result of more intensive glycaemic and BP control (Figure 4.3).

The relative risk for fatal coronary heart disease (CHD) in patients with type 2 diabetes compared with no diabetes is

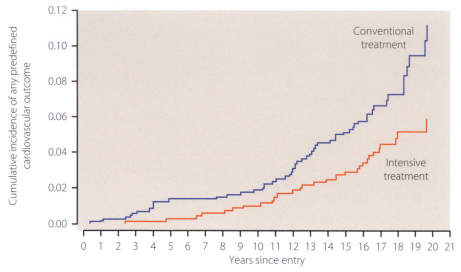

Figure 4.3 The long-term cardiovascular outcomes for patients with type 1 diabetes are improved by early intensive glycaemic control. Intensive control reduces the risk of any cardiovascular disease event by 42%. Adapted from the DCCT/EDIC Research Group. N Engl J Med 2005; 353: 2643–2653.

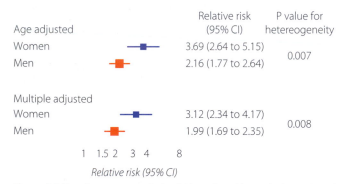

	Relative risk (95% CI)	P value for heterogeneity
Age adjusted		
Women	3.69 (2.64 to 5.15)	0.007
Men	2.16 (1.77 to 2.64)	
Multiple adjusted		
Women	3.12 (2.34 to 4.17)	0.008
Men	1.99 (1.69 to 2.35)	

Relative risk (95% CI)

Figure 4.4 Based on a meta-analysis of 22 studies, this graph shows the relative risks of fatal CHD in men and women with type 2 diabetes. Adapted from Huxley et al. BMJ 2006; 332: 73–76.

Table 4.2 The relative risk of ischaemic heart disease and stroke for every 1 mmol/L increase in fasting plasma glucose (FPG) concentration, even in the non-diabetic range, according to different age groups (after adjustment for confounding and regression dilution bias). FPG is a continuous variable in the global risk of mortality attributable to heart disease and stroke. From Danaei et al. Lancet 2006; 368: 1651–1659

	<60 years	60–69 years	≥70 years
Ischaemic heart disease	1.424	1.196	1.196
Stroke	1.360	1.284	1.081

significantly higher for women (3.5-fold increased risk) than for men (2.5-fold) (Figure 4.4). Patients with diabetes also have a worse prognosis following a cardiovascular event. For example, the relative risk of death after myocardial infarction is 2–3-fold higher in patients with diabetes compared with non-diabetics.

Cardiovascular mortality risk increases continuously with blood glucose concentrations starting at levels well below the current thresholds for defining diabetes or impaired fasting glycaemia. Based on population health surveys in 52 countries and a meta-analysis involving >200,000 subjects in the Asia-Pacific region, public health analysts have concluded that 21% of all deaths from ischaemic heart disease and 13% of deaths from stroke were attributable to higher than optimum blood glucose levels (Table 4.2).

Diabetes is a serious global health problem, and one that is going to become much worse. It already affects at least 5–7% of the world's population, and its prevalence is expected to increase from 171 million in 2000 to 366 million people by 2030; 90% of these people will have type 2 diabetes. Currently, there are 57 million people in the USA with prediabetes; most have the 'metabolic syndrome'.

Incidence of type 1 and type 2 diabetes and regional variations

An epidemic of obesity is driving the increased prevalence of type 2 diabetes (Figure 4.5), but the incidence of type 1 diabetes is also steadily increasing. If the present trends continue, there will be a doubling in the number of children in Europe with type 1 diabetes below the age of 5 years before 2020. An emerging dietary risk factor for type 1 diabetes is consumption of root vegetables (potatoes, carrots, etc.). In addition, placental transmission of viruses leading to type 1 diabetes (e.g. rubella) has been recognised. The genetic risk for type 1 diabetes is conferred mainly by HLA-DR and HLA-DQ haplotypes, but environmental

CASE HISTORY

A 66-year-old man of South Asian origin is admitted to hospital as an emergency with chest pain and acute (non-ST elevation) myocardial infarction. His only past medical history is of hypertension and obesity (BMI 33.8). He is a non-smoker and runs a newsagent shop. He takes lisinopril 10 mg daily. On talking to his wife, there is no known history of diabetes and he has not been previously tested. He takes little exercise. Admission blood tests show a random blood glucose of 21.6 mmol/L and HbA_{1c} 9.5%. He is treated with low molecular weight heparin and combination antiplatelet therapy, and blood glucose levels are controlled using a sliding scale IV insulin infusion. Subsequent investigations show that he has triple vessel disease, and he is referred for coronary artery bypass grafting. Blood sugar levels settle with metformin 850 mg bid, and he is seen by a dietitian.

Comment: This case illustrates a number of public health issues. Firstly, the elevated HbA_{1c} indicates that his diabetes has probably been present for some time; given that he has at least three risk factors for type 2 diabetes (hypertension, obesity and ethnicity), why was this not detected earlier? There is still some uncertainty about the benefits, costs and practicalities of screening. Secondly, late presentation and diagnosis usually means that more severe and more costly complications occur which could have been prevented. And thirdly, the South Asian population represents a particularly high-risk group in whom health inequalities often compound the clinical complications of diabetes.

LANDMARK CLINICAL TRIALS

Booth GL, Kapral M, Fung K, Tu J. Relation between age and cardiovascular disease in men and women with diabetes compared with non-diabetic people: a population-based retrospective cohort study. Lancet 2006; 368: 29–36.

Danaei G, Lawes C, Vander Hoorn S, et al. Global and regional mortality from ischaemic heart disease and stroke attributable to higher-than-optimum blood glucose concentration: comparative risk assessment. Lancet 2006; 368: 1651–1659.

Diabetes Prevention Program Research Group. Reduction in the incidence of type 2 diabetes with lifestyle intervention or metformin. N Engl J Med 2002; 346: 393–403.

Huxley R, Barzi F, Woodward M. Excess risk of fatal coronary heart disease associated with diabetes in men and women: meta-analysis of 37 prospective cohort studies. BMJ 2006; 332: 73–76.

Li G, Zhang P, Wang J, et al. The long-term effect of lifestyle interventions to prevent diabetes in the China Da Qing Diabetes Prevention study: a 20-year follow-up study. Lancet 2008; 371: 1783–1789.

Patterson CC, Dahlquist G, Gyurus E, et al. Incidence trends for childhood type 1 diabetes in Europe during 1989–2003 and predicted new cases 2005–2020: a multicentre prospective registration study. Lancet 2009; 373: 2027–2033.

Wild S, Roglic G, Green A, et al. Global prevalence of diabetes. Estimates for the year 2000 and projections for 2030. Diabet Care 2004; 27: 1047–1053.

Yang W, Lu J, Weng J, et al. Prevalence of diabetes among men and women in China. N Engl J Med 2010; 362: 1090–1101.

triggers are needed to induce islet autoimmunity in genetically predisposed individuals.

The frequency of diabetes is rising, especially in developing countries, where the lifestyle has changed from one based on traditional, agricultural subsistence to a westernised, urban culture. Readily available high-energy foods and physical inactivity lead to obesity, and to diabetes in these susceptible populations. Many diabetic patients in developing countries present late with serious infections or tissue complications. Diabetic emergencies have a high mortality. Practical difficulties in developing countries include lack of doctors, nurses and dietitians and shortages of drugs, including insulin (Figure 4.6). India and China are particularly affected by the type 2 diabetes epidemic. There are an estimated 40 million patients with diabetes in India alone, and available data suggest that the mean HbA_{1c} is high, at 9%.

In the UK and other Western countries, type 2 diabetes is increasing most rapidly among south Asian people living in urban communities (Figure 4.7). Their risk of developing type 2 diabetes is 4–6-fold higher, the disease occurs at an earlier age and the risk of renal and cardiovascular complications is much higher than for other ethnic groups. Overcoming health inequalities, and providing intensive multiple risk factor interventions, is a priority for this group of patients who require specialist medical and dietetic input.

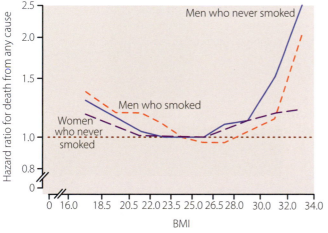

Figure 4.5 The relationship between Body Mass Index and the hazard ratio for death from any cause. Data for men according to smoking status, relative to females who never smoked, in a large Asian cohort study. Obesity carries an increased risk of several unwanted health outcomes, including diabetes, cardiovascular disease and certain forms of cancer. Adapted from Jee et al. N Engl J Med 2006; 355: 779–787.

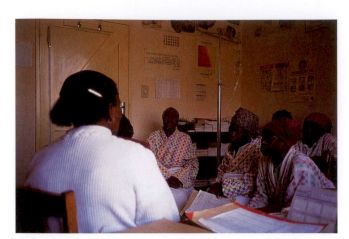

Figure 4.6 A morning education session, led by a nursing sister, at a hospital in Soweto, South Africa. All these patients had been admitted with diabetic emergencies in the previous 24 hours.

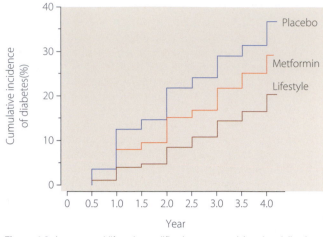

Figure 4.8 A structured lifestyle modification program (aimed at delivering >7% weight loss and 150 minutes of physical activity per week) is superior to drug treatment with metformin and placebo in diabetes prevention. Lifestyle intervention reduced the risk of type 2 diabetes by 58%. Adapted from Diabetes Prevention Study. N Engl J Med 2002; 346: 393–403.

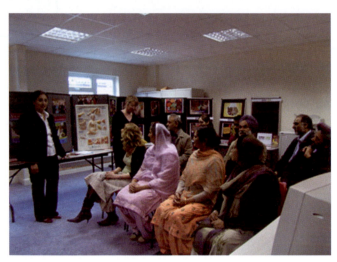

Figure 4.7 A structured diabetes education class for South Asians with type 2 diabetes.

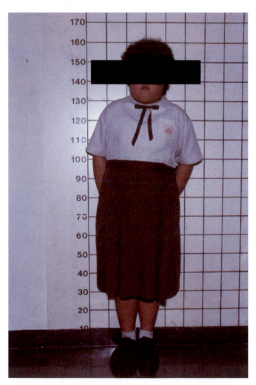

Figure 4.9 An 11-year-old girl from Hong Kong with type 2 diabetes. Note the marked truncal obesity.

Despite the rising incidence, costs and morbidity associated with diabetes, there is no clear policy in many countries for routine screening. A new primary care initiative in the UK recommends systematic assessment of cardiovascular risk among people aged 40–75 years, which includes testing for diabetes and impaired glucose tolerance (IGT) in high-risk groups. Adoption of HbA_{1c} for screening and diagnosis overcomes many of the practical limitations of fasting glucose and OGTT. Lifestyle modification is the most clinically effective and cost-effective intervention to prevent type 2 diabetes (Figure 4.8).

Traditionally, type 2 diabetes has been a disease of the middle aged and elderly, but the disease is now becoming a problem among adolescents and even children (Figure 4.9). A sedentary lifestyle and obesity are the main contributory factors, though many have a positive family history of type 2 diabetes. In some parts of the USA, type 2 diabetes now accounts for one-third of new cases of diabetes in adolescence.

KEY WEBSITES

- NHS Diabetes website: www.diabetes.nhs.uk/work-areas/ information/national-diabetes-public-health-info-group
- Diabetes National Service Framework: www.dh.gov.uk/en/Healthcare/ NationalServiceFrameworks/Diabetes/index.htm
- Diabetes information homepage of the US Centers for Disease Control and Prevention: www.cdc.gov/Diabetes/

FURTHER READING

Alexander GC, Sehgal N, Moloney R, Stafford R. National trends in treatment of type 2 diabetes mellitus, 1994–2007. Arch Intern Med 2008; 168: 2088–2094.

Bolen S. Systematic review: comparative effectiveness and safety of oral medications for type 2 diabetes mellitus. Ann Intern Med 2007; 147: 386–399.

Currie CJ, Peters JR, Tynan A, et al. Survival as a function of HbA_{1c} in people with type 2 diabetes: a retrospective cohort study. Lancet 2010; 375: 481–489.

Chowdhury T, Hitman GA. Diabetes care for South Asian patients: a special case. Lancet 2008; 371: 1728–1729.

Genuth S. The UKPDS and its global impact. Diabet Med 2008; 25(Suppl 2): 57–62.

Goyder EC. Screening for and prevention of type 2 diabetes. BMJ 2008; 336: 1140–1141.

Gray AM, Clarke P. The economic analyses of the UK Prospective Diabetes study. Diabetic Med 2008; 25(Suppl 2): 47–51.

Jee SH, Sull J, Park J, et al. Body-mass index and mortality in Korean men and women. N Engl J Med 2006; 355: 779–787.

McKinlay J, Marceau L. US public health and the 21st century: diabetes mellitus. Lancet 2000; 356: 757–761.

Selvin E, Steffes MW, Zhu H, et al. Glycated haemoglobin, diabetes and cardiovascular risk in nondiabetic adults. N Engl J Med 2010; 362: 800–811.

Trogdon JG, Hylands T. Nationally representative medical costs of diabetes by time since diagnosis. Diabetes Care 2008; 31: 2307–2311.

Normal physiology of insulin secretion and action

Islet structure and function

Insulin is synthesised in and secreted from the β cells within the islets of Langerhans in the pancreas. The normal pancreas has about 1 million islets, which constitute about 2–3% of the gland's mass. All of the islet cell types are derived embryologically from endodermal outgrowths of the fetal gut. The islets can be identified easily with various histological stains, such as haematoxylin and eosin (Figure 5.1), with which the cells react less intensely than does the surrounding exocrine tissue. The islets vary in size from a few dozen to several thousands of cells and are scattered irregularly throughout the exocrine pancreas.

The main cell types of the pancreatic islets are β cells that produce insulin, α cells that secrete glucagon, δ cells that produce somatostatin and PP cells that produce pancreatic polypeptide. The different cell types can be identified by immunostaining techniques, *in situ* hybridization for their hormone products (using nucleotide probes complementary to the target mRNA) and the electron microscope appearance of their secretory granules. The β cells are the most

numerous cell type and are located mainly in the core of the islet, while α and δ cells are located in the periphery (Figure 5.2).

Islet cells interact with each other through direct contact and through their products (e.g. glucagon stimulates insulin secretion and somatostatin inhibits insulin and glucagon

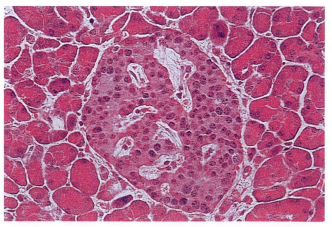

Figure 5.1 A section of normal pancreas stained with haematoxylin and eosin. As observed by Paul Langerhans, the islet in the centre is identified easily by its distinct morphology and lighter staining than that of the surrounding exocrine tissue (original magnification ×350).

Handbook of Diabetes, 4th edition. By © Rudy Bilous & Richard Donnelly. Published 2010 by Blackwell Publishing Ltd.

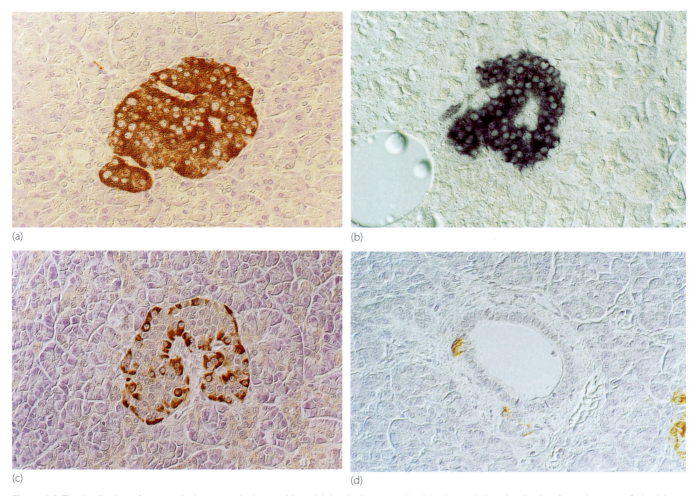

(a)   (b)

(c)   (d)

Figure 5.2 The localization of pancreatic hormones in human islets. (a) Insulin immunostained in the majority of cells that form the core of the islet (peroxidase–antiperoxidase immunostain with haematoxylin counterstain). (b) Insulin mRNA localized by *in situ* hybridization with a digoxigenin-labelled sequence of rat insulin cRNA (which cross-reacts fully with human insulin mRNA). (c) Peripherally located α cells immunostained with antibodies to pancreatic glucagon using the same method as for (a). (d) Weakly immunoreactive PP cells in the epithelium of a duct in the ventral portion of the pancreatic head. Magnifications approximately ×150.

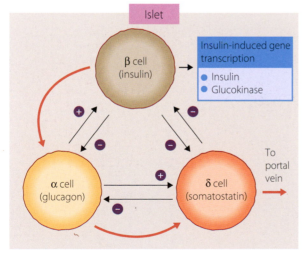

Figure 5.3 Potential interactions between the secretory products of the major islet cell types. Black arrows indicate paracrine stimulation or inhibition. The direction of blood flow within the islet is indicated by the red arrows.

secretion) (Figure 5.3). The blood flow within the islets is organised centrifugally so that the different cell types are supplied in the sequence β → α → δ. Insulin also has an 'autocrine' (self-regulating) effect that alters the transcription of insulin and glucokinase genes in the β cell.

The pancreatic islets are densely innervated with autonomic and peptidergic nerve fibres (Figure 5.4). Parasympathetic innervation from the vagus stimulates insulin release, while adrenergic sympathetic nerves inhibit insulin and stimulate glucagon secretion. Other nerves that originate within the pancreas contain peptides such as vasoactive intestinal peptide (VIP), which stimulates the release of all islet hormones, and neuropeptide Y (NPY) which inhibits insulin secretion. The overall importance of these neuropetides in controlling islet cell secretion remains unclear.

Pancreatic β cells may change in size, number and function during normal ageing and development (Figure 5.5). β cell mass is determined by the net effect of four independent

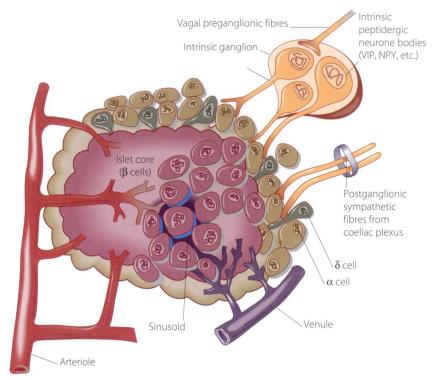

Figure 5.4 Structure of a pancreatic islet, showing the anatomical relationships between the four major endocrine cell types. NPY, neuropeptide Y; VIP, vasoactive intestinal polypeptide.

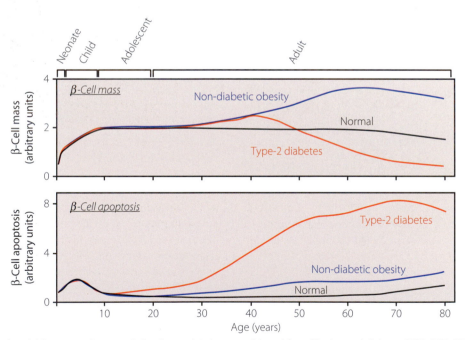

Figure 5.5 A hypothetical model for postnatal pancreatic β cell growth in humans. Adapted from Rhodes et al. Science 2005; 307: 380–384.

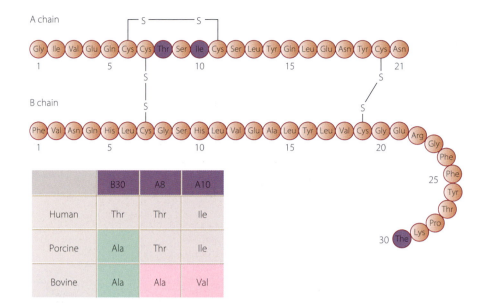

	B30	A8	A10
Human	Thr	Thr	Ile
Porcine	Ala	Thr	Ile
Bovine	Ala	Ala	Val

Figure 5.6 The primary structure (amino acid sequence) of human insulin. The highlighted residues are those that differ in porcine and bovine insulins, as shown in the inset.

CASE HISTORY

A 32-year-old woman develops impaired glucose tolerance at 34 weeks into her second pregnancy. She is managed with dietary modification, and the baby is delivered at 37 weeks. Her glucose tolerance returns to normal 6 weeks later. Her BMI is 31 kg/m², and her mother developed type 2 diabetes at the age of 55 years.

Comment: This woman had normal glucose tolerance prior to pregnancy, but the metabolic and endocrine changes associated with pregnancy resulted in transient impairment of glucose tolerance. This occurred because pancreatic insulin secretion was insufficient to compensate for increased insulin resistance as a result of pregnancy (on a background of obesity and a genetic predisposition). Genetic, dietary and endocrine factors affect β cell function. A history of gestational diabetes is a major risk factor for later development of type 2 diabetes in women.

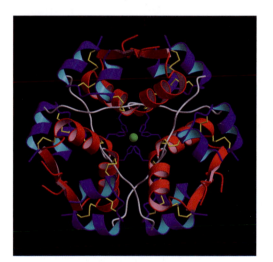

Figure 5.7 The double zinc insulin hexamer composed of three insulin dimers in a threefold symmetrical pattern.

mechanisms: (i) β cell replication (i.e. division of existing β cells), (ii) β cell size, (iii) β cell neogenesis (i.e. emergence of new β cells from pancreatic ductal epithelial cells) and (iv) β cell apoptosis. The contribution made by each of these processes is variable and may change at different stages of life.

Insulin synthesis and polypeptide structure

The insulin molecule consists of two polypeptide chains, linked by disulphide bridges; the A-chain contains 21 amino acids and the B-chain 30 amino acids. Human insulin differs from pig insulin (an animal insulin which was used exten-

sively for diabetes treatment prior to the 1990s) at only one amino acid position (B30) (Figure 5.6).

In dilute solution and in the circulation, insulin exists as a monomer of 6000 Da molecular weight. The tertiary (three-dimensional) structure of monomeric insulin consists of a hydrophobic core buried beneath a surface that is hydrophilic, except for two non-polar regions involved in the aggregation of the monomers into dimers and hexamers. In concentrated solution (such as in the insulin vial supplied by the pharmaceutical company for injection) and in crystals (such as in the insulin secretory granule), six monomers self-associate with two zinc ions to form a hexamer (Figure 5.7). This is of therapeutic importance because the slow absorption of native insulin from the subcutaneous tissue partly results

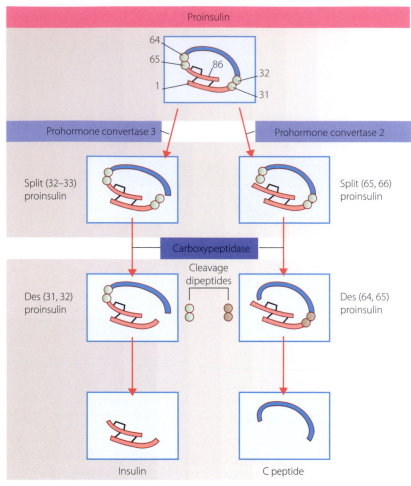

Figure 5.8 Insulin biosynthesis and processing. Proinsulin is cleaved on the C-terminal side of two dipeptides. The cleavage dipeptides are liberated, so yielding the 'split' proinsulin products and ultimately insulin and C-peptide.

LANDMARK CLINICAL TRIALS

Bell GI, Polonsky KS. Diabetes mellitus and genetically programmed defects in beta cell function. Nature 2001; 414: 788–791.

Bouatia-Naji N, Rocheleau G, van Lommel L, et al. A polymorphism within the G6PC2 gene is associated with fasting plasma glucose levels. Science 2008; 320: 1085–1088.

Dyachok O, Isakov Y, Sagetorp J, Tengholm A. Oscillations of cyclic AMP in hormone-stimulated insulin-secreting beta cells. Nature 2006; 439: 349–352.

Grimsby J, Sarabu R, Corbett W, et al. Allosteric activators of glucokinase: potential role in diabetes therapy. Science 2003; 301: 370–373.

Illies C, Gromada J, Fiume R, et al. Requirement of inositol pyrophosphates for full exocytotic capacity in pancreatic beta cells. Science 2007; 318: 1299–1302.

Lowell BB, Shulman GI. Mitochondrial dysfunction and type 2 diabetes. Science 2005; 307: 384–387.

Maechler P, Wollheim CB. Mitochondrial function in normal and diabetic beta cells. Nature 2001; 414: 807–812.

Marx J. Unravelling the causes of diabetes. Science 2002; 296: 686–689.

Poy MN, Eliasson L, Krutzfeldt J, et al. A pancreatic islet-specific microRNA regulates insulin secretion. Nature 2004; 432: 226–230.

Zhou Q, Brown J, Kanarek A, et al. In vivo reprogramming of adult pancreatic exocrine cells to beta cells. Nature 2008; 455: 627–632.

from the time taken for the hexameric insulin to dissociate into the smaller, more easily absorbed monomeric form.

Insulin is synthesised in the β cells from a single amino acid chain precursor molecule called proinsulin (Figure 5.8).

Synthesis begins with the formation of an even larger precursor, preproinsulin, which is cleaved by protease activity to proinsulin. The gene for preproinsulin (and therefore the 'gene for insulin') is located on chromosome 11. Proinsulin

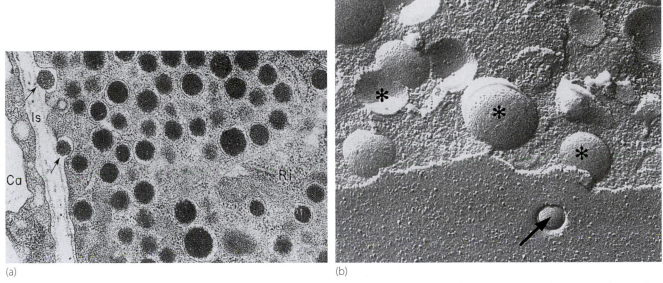

(a)   (b)

Figure 5.9 (a) Electron micrograph of insulin secretory granules in a pancreatic β cell and their secretion by exocytosis. Arrows show exocytosis occurring. Ca, capillary lumen; Is, interstitial space. (b) Freeze-fracture views of β cells that reveal the secretory granules in the cytoplasm (*asterisks*) and the granule content released by exocytosis at the cell membrane (*arrows*). Magnification: ×52,000. From Orci. Diabetologia 1974; 10: 163–187.

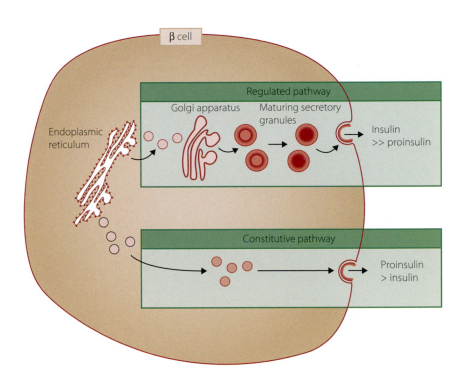

Figure 5.10 The regulated (normal) and constitutive (active in type 2 diabetes) pathways of insulin processing.

is packaged into vesicles in the Golgi apparatus of the β cell; in the maturing secretory granules that bud off it, proinsulin is converted by enzymes into insulin and connecting peptide (C-peptide).

Insulin and C-peptide are released from the β cell when the granules are transported ('translocated') to the cell surface and fuse with the plasma membrane (exocytosis) (Figure 5.9). Microtubules, formed of polymerised tubulin, probably provide the mechanical framework for granule transport, and microfilaments of actin, interacting with myosin and other motor proteins such as kinesin, may provide the motive force that propels the granules along the tubules. Although the actin cytoskeleton is a key mediator of biphasic insulin release, cyclic GTPases are involved in

F-actin reorganization in the islet β cell and play a crucial role in stimulus-secretion coupling.

This 'regulated pathway', with almost complete cleavage of proinsulin to insulin, normally carries about 95% of the β cell insulin production (Figure 5.10). In certain conditions, such as insulinoma and type 2 diabetes, an alternative 'constitutive' pathway operates, in which large amounts of unprocessed proinsulin and intermediate insulin precursors ('split proinsulins') are released directly from vesicles that originate in the endoplasmic reticulum.

Insulin secretion

Glucose is the main stimulator of insulin release from the β cell, which occurs in a characteristic biphasic pattern – an acute 'first phase' that lasts only a few minutes, followed by a sustained 'second phase' (Figure 5.11). The first phase of release involves the plasma membrane fusion of a small, readily releasable pool of granules; these granules discharge their contents in response to both nutrient and non-nutrient secretagogues. In contrast, second-phase insulin secretion is evoked exclusively by nutrients. The shape of the glucose–insulin dose–response curve is determined primarily by the activity of glucokinase, which governs the rate-limiting step for glucose metabolism in the β cell. Glucose levels below 5 mmol/L (90 mg/dL) do not affect insulin release; half-maximal stimulation occurs at about 8 mmol/L (144 mg/dL).

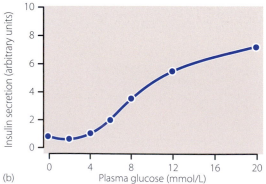

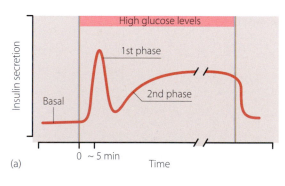

Figure 5.11 (a) The biphasic glucose-stimulated release of insulin from pancreatic islets. (b) The glucose–insulin dose–response curve for islets of Langerhans.

Glucose must be metabolised within the β cell to stimulate insulin secretion (Figure 5.12). It enters the β cell via the GLUT-2 transporter and is then phosphorylated by glucokinase, which acts as the 'glucose sensor' that couples insulin secretion to the prevailing glucose level. Glycolysis and mitochondrial metabolism produce adenosine triphosphate (ATP), which closes ATP-sensitive potassium (KATP) channels. This in turn causes depolarization of the β cell plasma membrane, which leads to an influx of extracellular calcium through voltage-gated channels in the membrane. The increase in cytosolic calcium triggers granule translocation and exocytosis. Sulphonylureas stimulate insulin secretion by binding to a component of the KATP channel (the sulphonylurea receptor, SUR-1) and closing it. The KATP channel is an octamer that consists of four K+-channel subunits (called Kir6.2) and four SUR-1 subunits.

The incretin effect

There is a significant difference between the insulin secretory response to oral glucose compared with the response to IV glucose – a phenomenon known as the 'incretin effect' (Figure 5.13). The incretin effect is mediated by gut-derived hormones, released in response to the ingestion of food, which augment glucose-stimulated insulin release. In particular, there are two incretin hormones: glucagon-like peptide-1 (GLP-1) and gastric inhibitory polypeptide (GIP). Both augment insulin secretion in a dose-dependent fashion. GLP-1 is secreted by L cells and GIP is secreted by K cells in the wall of the upper jejunum.

In patients with type 2 diabetes, GLP-1 secretion is diminished (Figure 5.14). However, in contrast to GIP, GLP-1 retains most of its insulinotropic activity. GIP secretion is maintained in type 2 diabetes, but its effect on the β cell is greatly reduced. GLP-1 also suppresses glucagon secretion from pancreatic α cells, and has effects on satiety and gastric emptying. There is also considerable interest in the trophic effects of GLP-1 on β cells.

Insulin receptor signalling

Insulin exerts its main biological effects by binding to a cell surface receptor, a glycoprotein that consists of two extracellular α subunits and two β subunits that span the cell membrane. The receptor has tyrosine kinase enzyme activity (residing in the β subunit), which is stimulated when insulin binds to the receptor. This enzyme phosphorylates tyrosine amino acid residues on various intracellular proteins, such as insulin receptor substrate (IRS)-1 and IRS-2, and the β subunit itself (Figure 5.15) (autophosphorylation). Tyrosine kinase activity is essential for insulin action.

Postreceptor signalling involves phosphorylation of a number of intracellular proteins that associate with the β subunit of the insulin receptor, including IRS-1 and IRS-2

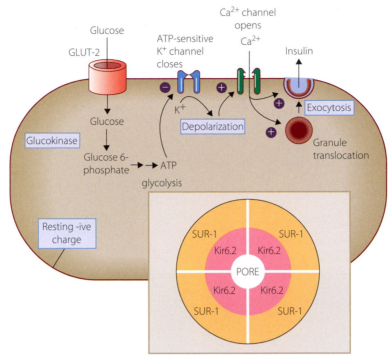

Figure 5.12 The mechanism of glucose-stimulated insulin secretion from the β cell. The structure of the KATP channel is shown in the inset.

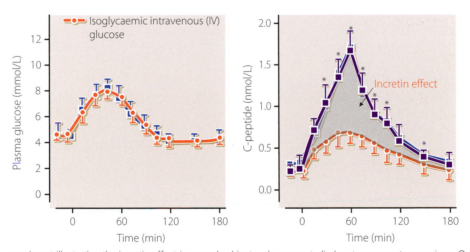

Figure 5.13 The classic experiment illustrating the incretin effect in normal subjects who were studied on two separate occasions. On one occasion, they were given an oral glucose load and on the second occasion an IV glucose bolus was administered in order to achieve identical venous plasma glucose concentration-time profiles on the two study days (left panel). The insulin secretory response (shown by C-peptide) was significantly greater after oral compared with IV glucose (right panel). Adapted from Nauck et al. J Clin Endocrinol Metab 1986; 63: 492–498.

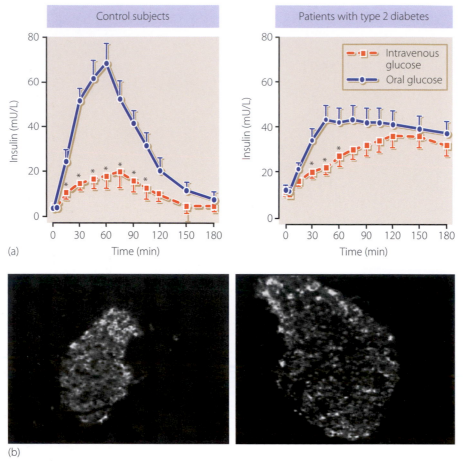

(a)

(b)

Figure 5.14 (a) The incretin effect is greatly diminished in patients with type 2 diabetes compared with normal subjects. This contributes to the impaired insulin secretory response observed in type 2 diabetes. (b) GLP-1 has a trophic effect on pancreatic islets . Shown here is an islet from a db/db mouse before (*left*) and after (*right*) 2 weeks treatment with synthetic GLP-1. Adapted from Stoffers et al. Diabetes 2000; 49: 741–748.

(Figure 5.16). Phosphorylated tyrosine residues on these proteins act as docking sites for the non-covalent binding of proteins with specific 'SH2' domains, such as phospatidyli-nositol 3-kinase (PI 3-kinase), Grb2 and phosphotyrosine phosphatase (SHP2). Binding of Grb2 to IRS-1 initiates a cascade that eventually activates nuclear transcription factors via activation of the protein Ras and mitogen-acti-vated protein (MAP) kinase. IRS–PI 3-kinase binding gener-ates phospholipids that modulate other specific kinases and regulate responses such as glucose transport, and protein and glycogen synthesis.

GLUT transporters

Glucose is transported into cells by a family of specialised transporter proteins called glucose transporters (GLUTs) (Figure 5.17). The process of glucose uptake is energy inde-pendent. The best characterised GLUTs are:

- GLUT-1: ubiquitously expressed and probably mediates basal, non-insulin mediated glucose uptake
- GLUT-2: present in the islet β cell, and also in the liver,

intestine and kidney. Together with glucokinase, it forms the β cell's glucose sensor and, because it has a high Km, allows glucose to enter the β cell at a rate proportional to the extracellular glucose level
- GLUT-3: together with GLUT-1, involved in non-insulin mediated uptake of glucose into the brain
- GLUT-4: responsible for insulin-stimulated glucose uptake in muscle and adipose tissue, and thus the classic hypogly-caemic action of insulin
- GLUT-8: important in blastocyst development
- GLUT-9 and 10: unclear functional significance.

Most of the other GLUTs are present at the cell surface, but in the basal state GLUT-4 is sequestered within vesicles in the cytoplasm. Insulin causes the vesicles to be translocated to the cell surface, where they fuse with the membrane and the inserted GLUT-4 unit functions as a pore that allows glucose entry into the cell. The process is reversible: when insulin levels fall, the plasma membrane GLUT-4 is removed by endocytosis and recycled back to intracellular vesicles for storage (Figure 5.18).

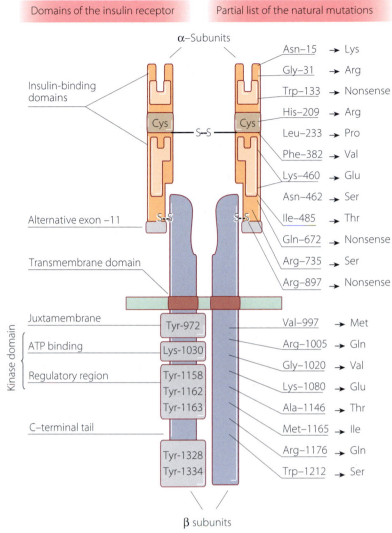

Figure 5.15 The insulin receptor and its structural domains. Many mutations have been discovered in the insulin receptor, some of which interfere with insulin's action and can cause insulin resistance; examples are shown in the right column.

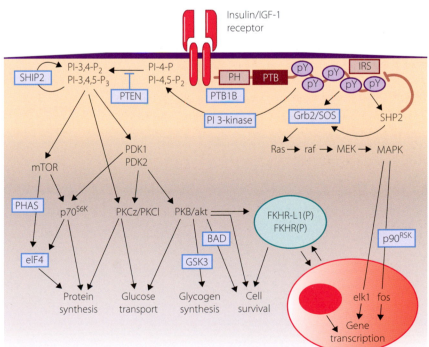

Figure 5.16 The insulin signalling cascade. Insulin binding and autophosphorylation of the insulin (and IGF-1) receptor results in binding of the IRS-1 protein to the β subunit of the insulin receptor via the IRS phosphotyrosine-binding domain (PTB). There is then phosphorylation of a number of tyrosine residues (pY) at the C-terminus of the IRS proteins. This leads to recruitment and binding of downstream signalling proteins, such as PI-3 kinase, Grb2 and SHP2.

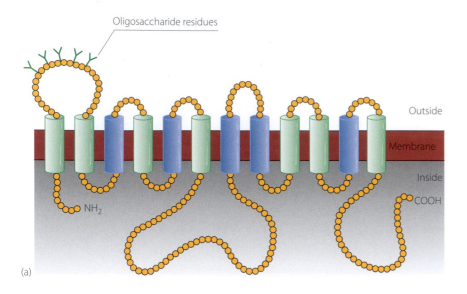

Oligosaccharide residues

Outside

Membrane

Inside

NH_2

COOH

(a)

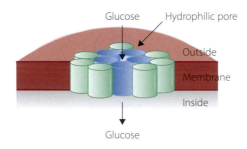

Glucose   Hydrophilic pore

Outside

Membrane

Inside

Glucose

(b)

Figure 5.17 (a) The structure of a typical glucose transporter (GLUT). (b) The intramembrane domains pack together to form a central hydrophilic channel through which glucose passes.

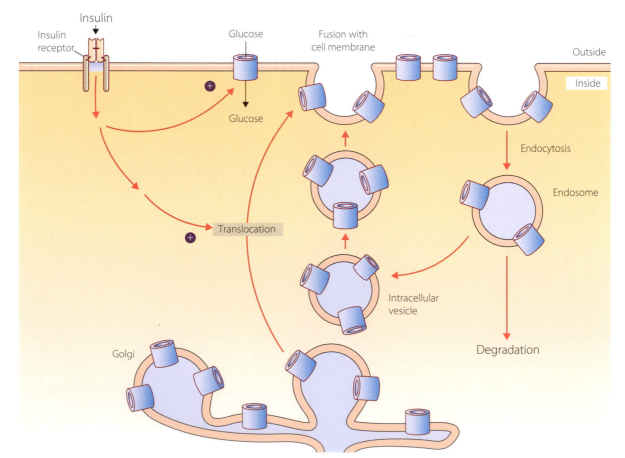

Insulin

Insulin receptor

Glucose

Fusion with cell membrane

Outside

Inside

Glucose

Endocytosis

Endosome

+

+

Translocation

Intracellular vesicle

Degradation

Golgi

Figure 5.18 Insulin regulation of glucose transport into cells.

In normal subjects, blood glucose concentrations are maintained within relatively narrow limits at around 5 mmol/L (90 mg/dL) (Figure 5.19). This is achieved by a balance between glucose entry into the circulation from the liver and from intestinal absorption, and glucose uptake into the peripheral tissues such as muscle and adipose tissue. Insulin is secreted at a low, basal level in the non-fed state, with increased, stimulated levels at mealtimes.

At rest in the fasting state, the brain consumes about 80% of the glucose utilised by the whole body, but brain glucose uptake is not regulated by insulin. Glucose is the main fuel for the brain, so that brain function critically depends on the maintenance of normal blood glucose levels.

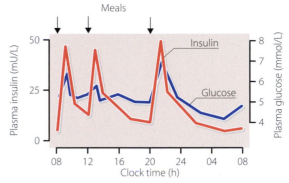

Figure 5.19 Profiles of plasma glucose and insulin concentrations in individuals without diabetes.

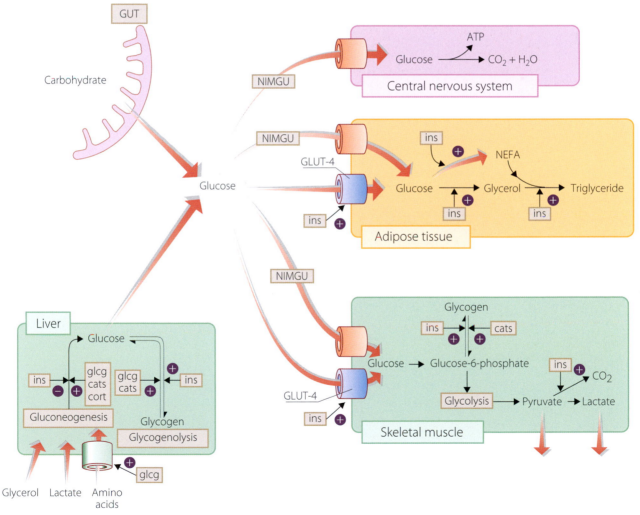

Figure 5.20 Overview of carbohydrate metabolism. cats, catecholamines; cort, cortisol; glcg, glucagon; ins, insulin; NIMGU, non-insulin mediated glucose uptake.

Insulin lowers glucose levels partly by suppressing glucose output from the liver, both by inhibiting glycogen breakdown (glycogenolysis) and by inhibiting gluconeogenesis (i.e. the formation of 'new' glucose from sources such as glycerol, lactate and amino acids, like alanine). Relatively low concentrations of insulin are needed to suppress hepatic glucose output in this way, such as occur with basal insulin secretion between meals and at night. With much higher insulin levels after meals, GLUT-4 mediated glucose uptake into the periphery is stimulated.

KEY WEBSITES

- www.vivo.colostate.edu/hbooks/pathphys/endocrine/pancreas/index.html
- www.accessmedicine.com/content.aspx?aid=2090245

FURTHER READING

Danial NN, Walensky L, Zhang C, et al. Dual role of proapoptotic BAD in insulin secretion and beta cell survival. Nat Med 2008; 14: 144–153.

Gauthier BR, Wollheim CB. MicroRNAs: 'ribo-regulators' of glucose homeostasis. Nat Med 2006; 12: 36–38.

Hou JC, Min L, Pessin J. Insulin granule biogenesis, trafficking and exocytosis. Vitam Horm 2009; 80: 473–506.

Kahn A. Converting hepatocytes to beta cells – a new approach for diabetes. Nat Med 2000; 6: 505–506.

Mello CC. Micromanaging insulin secretion. Nat Med 2004; 10: 1297–1298.

Moore A. Advances in beta cell imaging. Eur J Radiol 2009; 70: 254–257.

Rhodes CJ. Type 2 diabetes – a matter of β-cell life and death? Science 2005; 307: 380–384.

Tuttle RL, Gill N, Pugh W, et al. Regulation of pancreatic beta cell growth and survival by the serine/threonine protein kinase Akt1/PKBalpha. Nat Med 2001; 7: 1133–1137.

Wang Z, et al. Mechanisms of biphasic insulin-granule exocytosis – roles of the cytoskeleton, small GTPases and SNARE proteins. J Cell Science 2009; 122: 893–903.

Chapter 6

Epidemiology and aetiology of type 1 diabetes

KEY POINTS

- Type 1 diabetes is one of a number of autoimmune endocrine diseases with a genetic and familial basis, although the majority of cases occur sporadically.
- Incidence rates vary from <5 to >40 per 100,000, generally being highest in northern latitudes.
- These rates are increasing more rapidly than can be explained by genetic factors alone.
- Environmental factors such as viruses and diet are responsible for some of the increase.

The most common cause of type 1 diabetes (over 90% of cases) is T cell-mediated autoimmune destruction of the islet β cells leading to a failure of insulin production. The exact aetiology is complex and still imperfectly understood. However, it is probable that environmental factors trigger the onset of diabetes in individuals with an inherited predisposition. Unless insulin replacement is given, absolute insulin deficiency will result in hyperglycaemia and ketoacidosis, which is the biochemical hallmark of type 1 diabetes.

There is a striking variation in the incidence of type 1 diabetes between and within populations, with high frequencies in Finland (49 cases/100,000/year) and Sweden (32/100,000/year), and low frequencies in areas of China and Venezuela (both 0.1/100,000/year) and the Ukraine (1/100,000/year). Marked differences also occur within the same country: the incidence in Sardinia (37/100,000/year) is 3–5 times that of mainland Italy. These differences in frequency suggest that environmental and/or ethnic–genetic factors may influence the onset of the disease.

The geographical variation within Europe has been highlighted by the EURODIAB epidemiology study. This survey found a 10-fold difference in the incidence of type 1 diabetes between Finland and Macedonia. The incidence generally falls along a north–south gradient, but Sardinia is a notable 'hot spot' with a much higher frequency than the surrounding Mediterranean areas. Interestingly, there are also different incidences in genetically similar countries such as Finland and Estonia, or Norway and Iceland. Moreover, the most recent report suggests an overall annual rate of increase

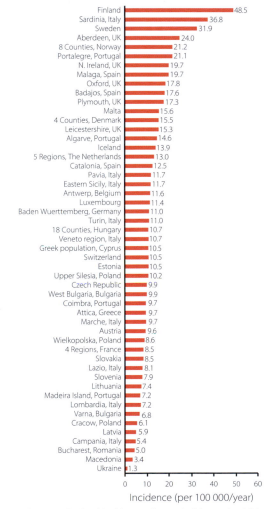

Figure 6.1 Age-standardised incidence of type 1 diabetes in children 14 years of age (per 100,000 per year). From Pickup & Williams. *Textbook of Diabetes*, 3rd edition. Blackwell Publishing Ltd, 2003.

Handbook of Diabetes, 4th edition. By © Rudy Bilous & Richard Donnelly. Published 2010 by Blackwell Publishing Ltd.

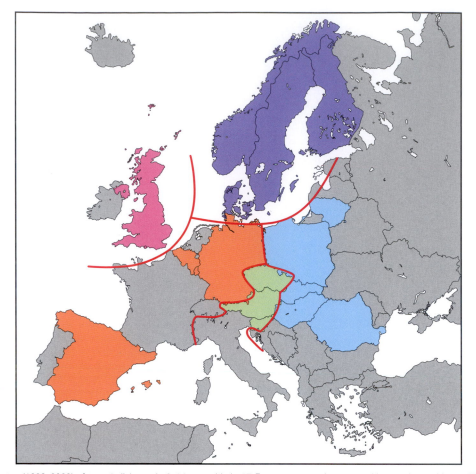

Figure 6.2 Incidence rates (1999–2003) of type 1 diabetes in 0–14 year olds in 17 European countries grouped into regions with roughly homogeneous rates. Purple 22.9–52.6/100,000; pink 22.4–29.8/100,000; orange 13–18.3/100,000; green 11.1–17.2/100,000; and blue 11.3–13.6/100,000. Reproduced from Patterson et al. Lancet 2009; 373: 2027–2033).

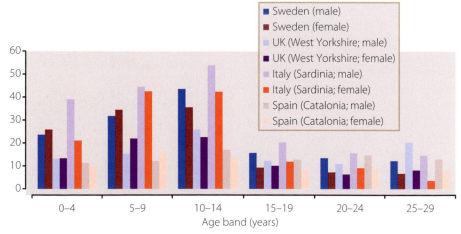

Figure 6.3 Incidence rates for type 1 diabetes in quintile age ranges 0–29 years in four countries in Europe in 1996–7. Note different rates in Catalonia and Sardinia despite a similar geographical latitude; and persistent male preponderance in all groups, especially aged 10–14 years. Data from *Diabetes Atlas*, 3rd edn.

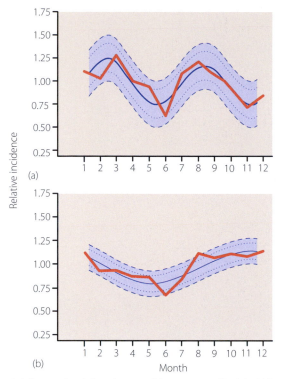

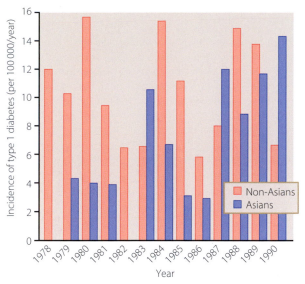

Figure 6.5 Evidence of environmental factors: incidence of type 1 diabetes in children from Asian families who moved to Bradford, UK, compared to non-Asian local UK children. Data from Bodansky et al. BMJ 1992; 304: 1020–1022.

Figure 6.4 Seasonal variation of type 1 diabetes among Finnish children (a) 0–9 years of age, (b) 10–14 years of age during 1983–92. (The observed monthly variation in incidence is the solid line with dots.) The inner interval is the 95% confidence interval (CI) for the observed seasonal variation and the outer interval is the 95% CI for the estimated seasonal variation. Data from Padaiga et al. Diabetic Med 1999; 16: 1–8.

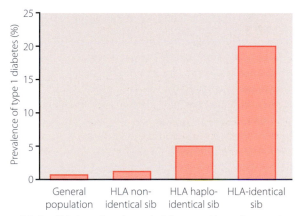

Figure 6.6 Familial clustering of type 1 diabetes: evidence for genetic factors in the aetiology. From Pickup & Williams. *Textbook of Diabetes*, 3rd edition. Blackwell Publishing Ltd, 2003.

in incidence in children aged below 15 years of 3.9% (range 0.6–9.3%). Prevalence is predicted to rise from 94,000 (2005) to 160,000 in 2020 in Europe. This suggests that environmental influences may predominate over genetic susceptibility in causing or triggering the disease.

Further evidence for environmental influences comes from studies that show a seasonal variation in the onset of type 1 diabetes in some populations, with the highest frequency in the colder autumn and winter months (Figure 6.4). This is often thought to reflect seasonal exposure to viruses, but food or chemicals might also be involved.

People who have migrated from an area of low to an area of high incidence for type 1 diabetes seem to adopt the same level of risk as the population to which they move. For example, children of Asian families (from the Indian subcontinent and Tanzania) who moved to the UK traditionally have a low frequency of type 1 diabetes but now have a rising incidence of the disease, which is approaching that of the indigenous population (Figure 6.5).

Familial clustering of type 1 diabetes provides evidence for complex genetic factors in its aetiology (Figure 6.6). In (European) siblings of children with type 1 diabetes, 5–6% have developed type 1 diabetes by the age of 15 years and

CASE HISTORY

A 4-year-old boy whose mother has had type 1 diabetes since age 13 years developed thirst, polyuria, hyperphagia and weight loss shortly after recovering from a head cold. His mother tested his capillary blood glucose with her own meter and found it to be 25.3 mmol/L. His birth weight was 4.1 kg and he was bottle fed with cow's milk from birth.

Comment: This case illustrates several cardinal features of type 1 diabetes. A positive family history, age of onset <5 years, symptoms beginning after a minor infection, and early exposure to cow's milk. Birth weight >4 kg is linked to type 2 diabetes in some populations.

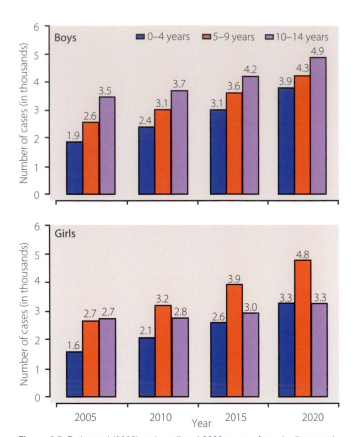

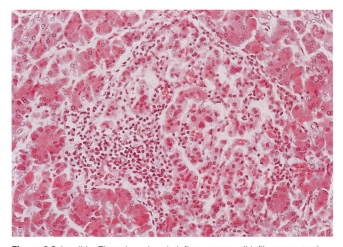

Figure 6.7 Estimated (2005) and predicted 2020 cases of newly diagnosed type 1 diabetes by age and sex for Europe excluding Belarus, the Russian Federation, Ukraine, Moldova and Albania using Poisson regression modelling. Reproduced from Patterson et al. Lancet 2009; 373: 2027–2033.

20% have diabetes if they are human leukocyte antigen (HLA) identical, compared with the population frequency of about 0.4%. However, only 10–15% of type 1 diabetes occurs in families with the disease ('multiplex') and most cases are said to be 'sporadic'. The chance of a child developing type 1 diabetes is around 5% if one parent is affected or 15% if both have the condition. The risk is greater if the father is affected and there is also a small male preponderance in overall prevalence. The reasons for these sex differences remain unknown.

The incidence of type 1 diabetes is increasing in many countries. In Europe, the overall increase is 3.4% per year, but the increase is particularly notable in those diagnosed under the age of 5 years, where it is 6.3% per year and total numbers are likely to double by 2020 (Figure 6.7). Based on these figures, the prevalence of type 1 diabetes may be 70% higher in 2020 than in 1989. This sharp rise in frequency over a short period of time suggests changing environmental factors that operate in early life, as genetic factors would take much longer over several generations to make an impact.

Aetiology
Autoimmunity

Evidence for autoimmunity in the pathogenesis of type 1 diabetes comes from postmortem studies in patients who have died shortly after presentation and pancreatic biopsies from living patients. They have revealed a chronic inflammatory mononuclear cell infiltrate ('insulitis') (Figure 6.8) associated with the residual β cells in the islets of recently diagnosed type 1 diabetic patients. The infiltrate consists of

Figure 6.8 Insulitis. There is a chronic inflammatory cell infiltrate centred on this islet. Haematoxylin–eosin stain, original magnification ×300.

T cell lymphocytes and macrophages. Later in the disease, there is complete loss of β cells, while the other islet cell types (α, δ and PP cells) all survive.

A major marker of insulitis is the presence of four circulating islet-related autoantibodies in patients with newly diagnosed type 1 diabetes; islet cells (ICAs), insulin molecule (IAAs), tyrosine phosphatase (IA-2) and glutamic acid decarboxylase (GAD) antibodies. However, not all those with islet autoantibodies go on to develop diabetes, which suggests that insulitis does not necessarily progress to critical β cell damage. Type 1 diabetes is manifest clinically after a prodromal period of months or years, during which immunological abnormalities, such as circulating islet autoantibodies, can be detected, even though normoglycaemia is maintained.

In family studies, positivity to three or more autoantibodies confers a risk of developing type 1 diabetes of 60–100% over 5–10 years. Single positivity carries a much lower positive predictive value.

The autoimmune basis for type 1 diabetes is also suggested by its association with other diseases such as hypothyroidism, Graves' disease, pernicious anaemia and Addison's disease which are all associated with organ-specific autoantibodies (Box 6.1). Up to 30% of people with type 1 diabetes have autoimmune thyroid disease.

The detection of ICAs and GAD antibodies in older persons with type 2 diabetes in Finland and the UKPDS, who were shown subsequently to be more likely to require insulin therapy, has led to the concept of latent autoimmune diabetes of adults (LADA). However, this concept has been challenged. Although GAD positivity had a specificity of 94.6% for early insulin use in the UKPDS, its sensitivity was only 37.9%. Moreover, the positive predictive value for GAD-positive antibodies was only 50.8% (i.e. only half of those positive went on to need insulin). Furthermore, people with LADA had a similar pattern of HLA haplotype (see below) as those developing type 1 diabetes in childhood. It is likely therefore that as LADA patients have some but not all of the immunological markers of type 1 diabetes of childhood, they represent part of a spectrum of autoimmune disease rather than a separate entity in their own right.

Genetics

Genetic susceptibility to type 1 diabetes is most closely associated with HLA genes that lie within the major histocompatibility complex (MHC) region on the short arm of chromosome 6 (now called the IDDM1 locus). HLAs are cell surface glycoproteins that show extreme variability through polymorphisms in the genes that code for them. Both high- and low-risk HLA haplotypes have been identified. HLA DR/4, DQA1* 0301–DQB1* 0302 and DQA1* 0501–DQB1* 0201 account for over 50% of genetic susceptibility; whereas DQA1* 0102–DQB1* 0602 and DRB1* 1401 are protective.

Class II HLAs (HLA-D) play a key role in presenting foreign and self-antigens to T-helper lymphocytes and therefore in initiating the autoimmune process (Figure 6.11). Polymorphisms in the DQB1 gene that result in amino acid substitutions in the class II antigens may affect the ability to accept and present autoantigens derived from the β cell. This is a critical step in 'arming' T lymphocytes, which initiate the immune attack against the β cells.

Over 20 regions of the human genome are associated with type 1 diabetes, but most make only a minor contribution. IDDM2 corresponds to the insulin VNTR gene locus on

---

Box 6.1 Autoimmune disorders associated with type 1 diabetes

- Addison's disease
- Graves' disease
- Hypothyroidism
- Hypogonadism
- Pernicious anaemia
- Vitiligo
- Autoimmune polyglandular syndromes, types 1 and 2
- Coeliac disease

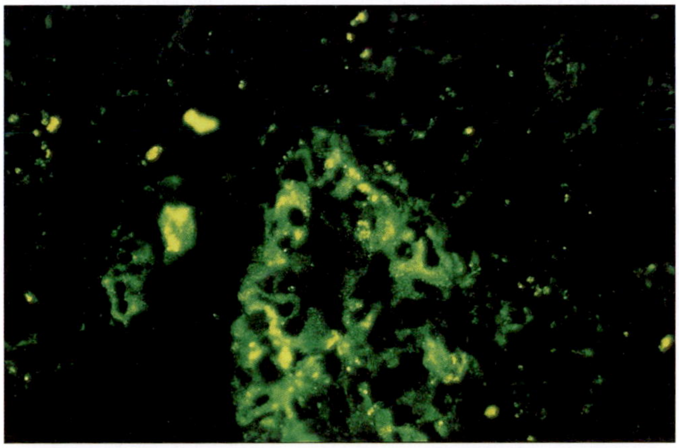

Figure 6.9 ICA demonstrated by indirect immunofluorescence in a frozen section of human pancreas.

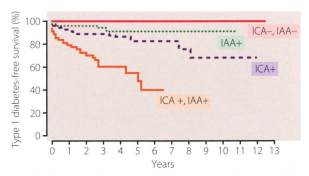

Figure 6.10 The probability of remaining free of type 1 diabetes in 4694 non-diabetic relatives of patients with type 1 diabetes. Disease-free survival was dependent on the presence of islet-related antibodies, the greatest risk being when both islet cell antibodies (ICAs) and insulin autoantibodies (IAAs) were present together. Data from Krischer et al. J Clin Endocrinol Metab 1993: 77:743–749.

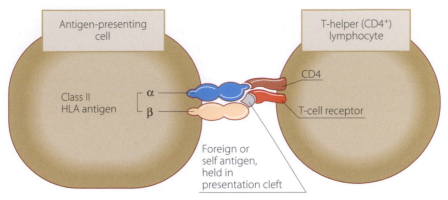

Figure 6.11 Antigen associated with class II HLA is presented to T cells.

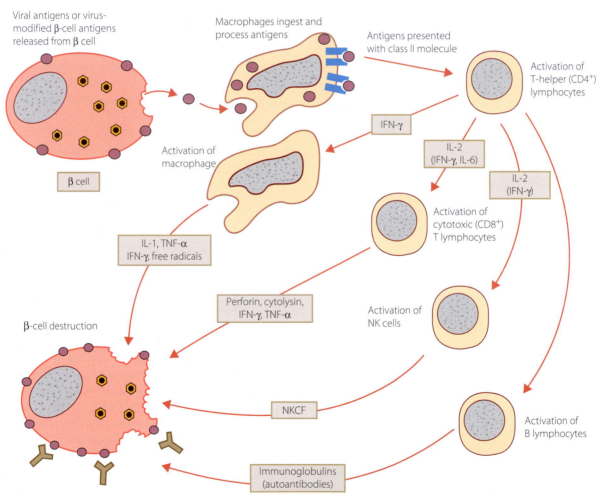

Figure 6.12 Hypothetical scheme that shows ways in which viruses could initiate an autoimmune attack on β cells. Some viruses (e.g. retroviruses and rubella virus) may induce β cells to express viral (foreign) antigens or render an endogenous β cell antigen immunogenic. Viral antigens released from β cells during normal β cell turnover might be processed by macrophages and presented to T-helper lymphocytes (CD4+) associated with HLA class II antigens. Activated T lymphocytes then secrete interleukin (IL)-2 and other cytokines that activate other immune cells. B lymphocytes produce immunoglobulins against the viral antigens, while activated natural killer (NK) cells and cytotoxic (CD8+) lymphocytes cause destruction of β cells that carry the viral antigens. Macrophages, activated by interferon-γ (IFN-γ), also participate in the destruction of the target cells. NKCF, natural killer cell factor; TNF, tumour necrosis factor.

chromosome 11, has a smaller effect than IDDM1 and acts independently. Together with IDDM 12 (CTLA-4), it contributes around 15% of the genetic risk. The other 17 genes individually contribute little. The predisposing polymorphism in the IDDM 2 gene and how it influences the disease has yet to be determined.

Environmental and maternal factors

Although genetic factors are undoubtedly important, the relatively low concordance of <50% in monozygotic twins together with the rapidly increasing incidence rates for type 1 diabetes at a younger age strongly suggest that external or environmental factors are playing a part. Much of the evidence that links environmental factors with the aetiology of type 1 diabetes is circumstantial, based upon epidemiology and animal research. The factors most often implicated are viruses, and diet and toxins, but a number of other influences, such as early feeding with cow's milk and psychological stress, are being investigated.

Recent meta-analyses and pooled cohort studies have shown a link to birth weight (a 7% increase in risk for every 1 kg in weight); Caesarean section (a 20% increase); and maternal age (5% increase for each 5 years). These associations remain unexplained.

Viruses

The viruses that have been implicated in the development of human diabetes have been deduced from temporal and geographical associations with a known infection. For example, mumps can cause pancreatitis and occasionally precedes the development of type 1 diabetes in children. Intrauterine rubella infection induces diabetes in up to 20% of affected children. Many people with recent-onset type 1 diabetes have serological or clinical evidence of coxsackie B virus infection, particularly the B4 serotype. Marked islet β cell damage has been detected in children who died from coxsackie B virus infection.

In a few cases, coxsackie viral antigens have been isolated in islets postmortem, and viruses isolated from the pancreas have been shown to induce diabetes in susceptible mouse strains. Electron microscopy of the pancreas in some subjects who died shortly after the onset of type 1 diabetes identified retrovirus-like particles within the β cells, associated with insulitis.

Viruses may target the β cells and destroy them directly through a cytolytic effect or by triggering an autoimmune attack (Figure 6.12). Autoimmune mechanisms may include 'molecular mimicry'; that is, immune responses against a viral antigen that cross-react with a β cell antigen (e.g. a coxsackie B4 protein (P2-C) has sequence homology with GAD, an established autoantigen in the β cell). Also, anti-insulin antibodies from type 1 diabetic patients cross-react with the retroviral p73 antigen in about 75% of cases.

Alternatively, viral damage may release sequestered islet antigens and thus restimulate resting autoreactive T cells, previously sensitised against β cell antigens ('bystander activation'). Persistent viral infection could also stimulate interferon-α synthesis and hyperexpression of HLA class I antigens, and the secretion of chemokines that recruit activated macrophages and cytotoxic T cells.

Apoptosis

One model of β cell destruction is via the process of apoptosis or programmed cell death (Figure 6.13). This is effected by the activation of cellular caspases triggered by several means, including the interaction of cell surface Fas (the death-signalling molecule) with its ligand FasL on the surface of infiltrating cells. Other factors that induce apoptosis include macrophage derived nitric oxide (NO) and toxic free radicals, and disruption of the cell membrane by perforin and granzyme B produced by cytotoxic T cells. T cell cytokines (e.g. interleukin-1, tumour necrosis factor-α, interferon-γ) upregulate Fas and FasL and induce NO and toxic free radicals.

Dietary factors

Wheat gluten is a potent diabetogen in animal models of type 1 diabetes (BB rats and NOD mice; see below), and 5–10% of patients with type 1 diabetes have gluten-sensitive enteropathy (coeliac disease). Recent studies have demonstrated that patients with type 1 diabetes and coeliac disease share disease-specific alleles. Wheat may induce subclinical gut inflammation and enhanced gut permeability to lumen antigens in some patients with type 1 diabetes, which may lead to a breakdown in tolerance for dietary proteins. Other possible diabetogenic factors in diet include N-nitroso compounds, speculatively implicated in Icelandic smoked meat, which was a common dietary constituent in winter months.

It has been suggested that early weaning and introduction of cow's milk may trigger type 1 diabetes, but this remains controversial. Surveys have shown associations between both the consumption of milk protein and a low prevalence of breastfeeding with the incidence of type 1 diabetes in different countries (Figure 6.14). It is hypothesised that antibodies against bovine serum albumin may cross-react with an islet antigen (ICA69). The studies are inconsistent, perhaps because of variations in milk composition or the existence of a subset of milk-sensitive, diabetes-prone people. Immune tolerance to insulin might also be compromised by cow's milk, which contains much less insulin than human milk.

Toxins

The notion that there may be environmental β cell toxins is supported by the existence of chemicals that cause an insulin-dependent type of diabetes in animals. Examples are

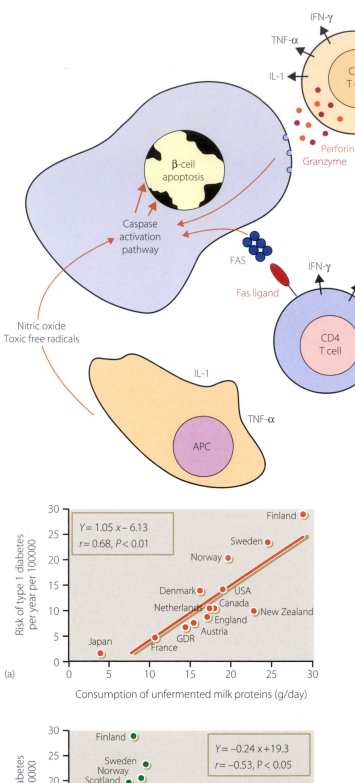

Figure 6.13 Proposed mechanisms of β cell death. B cells die through a process known as apoptosis, characterised by condensation and fragmentation of nuclear chromatin, loss of cytoplasm and expression of surface receptors that signal macrophages to ingest the apoptotic cell. Apoptosis is effected by activation of the caspase pathway.

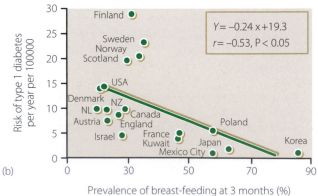

Figure 6.14 The relationship between risk of type 1 diabetes and (a) the consumption of milk protein and (b) the prevalence of breastfeeding in different countries. Data from Sandler. Abstracts of Uppsala Dissertations from the Faculty of Medicine, University of Uppsala, Sweden, 1983.

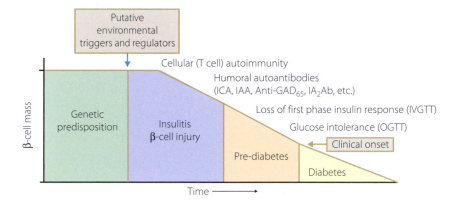

Figure 6.15 Depiction of the evolution of type 1 diabetes.

alloxan and streptozocin, both of which damage the β cell at several sites, including membrane disruption, enzyme interaction (e.g. with glucokinase) and DNA fragmentation. The rat poison vacor causes type 1 diabetes in humans, possibly because it has a similar action to streptozocin.

Animal models

Spontaneous diabetes that resembles type 1 diabetes in humans occurs in some animals, notably the BioBreeding (BB) rat and the non-obese diabetic (NOD) mouse. These 'animal models' have many of the same characteristics as human autoimmune diabetes, including a genetic predisposition, MHC association, insulitis, circulating islet cell surface and GAD autoantibodies, a long prediabetic period that precedes overt hyperglycaemia and environmental factors that trigger or accelerate the appearance of diabetes, such as wheat and cow's milk proteins.

Hygiene hypothesis

The increasing incidence of atopy as well as early-onset type 1 diabetes in Western societies may be a consequence of a lack of exposure to common pathogens such as mycobacteria, lactobacilli and helminth worms. Chronic exposure might include a more tolerant T cell response to antigens, while a cleaner, more sterile early environment would result in an exaggerated response. This hypothesis has increasing supportive associative data but remains unproven.

Combined model

One model of the evolution of type 1 diabetes is that individuals destined to develop the disease are born with genes that confer predisposition and they outweigh any genes with protective effects (Figure 6.15). Environmental factors then act as triggers of the T cell-mediated autoimmune destructive process, which results in insulitis, β cell injury and loss of β cell mass. As β cell function declines, there is loss of the first-phase insulin response to intravenous glucose, subsequent glucose intolerance (pre-diabetes) and eventually the clinical onset of overt diabetes. An alternative view is that there is a chronic interaction between genetic susceptibility, cumulative exposure to environmental factors and immune regulatory processes over the entire period until a critical loss of β cell mass results in insulin deficiency and hyperglycaemia. These events are assumed to proceed more rapidly in children.

FURTHER READING

Daneman D. Type 1 diabetes. Lancet 2006; 367: 847–858.
Gale EAM. The discovery of type 1 diabetes. Diabetes 2001; 50: 217–226.
Gale EAM. Latent autoimmune diabetes in adults: a guide for the perplexed. Diabetologia 2005; 48: 2195–2199.
Gale EAM. Maternal age and diabetes in childhood. BMJ 2010; 340: 436.
International Diabetes Federation. *Diabetes Atlas*, 4th edn. Brussels: International Diabetes Federation, 2009.
No authors listed. Type 1 and type 2 diabetes: less apart than apparent? Proceedings of the Sixth Servier-IGIS Symposium. Diabetes 2005; 54(Suppl 2): S1–S159.
Patterson CC, Dahlquist GG, Gyurus E, Green A, Soltesz G and the EURODIAB Study Group. Incidence trends for childhood type 1 diabetes in Europe during 1989–2003 and predicted new cases 2005–20: a multicentre prospective registration study. Lancet 2009; 373: 2027–2033.

Epidemiology and aetiology of type 2 diabetes

KEY POINTS

- Type 2 diabetes prevalence is set to increase to around 380 million persons worldwide by 2025, with the highest rates in the Eastern Mediterranean and Middle East, North and South America.
- Rates are also higher in urban compared to rural populations and are increasing dramatically in younger age groups, particularly adolescents.
- Obesity is closely linked to development of type 2 diabetes through its association with insulin resistance, partly mediated by

hormones and cytokines such as adiponectin, tumour necrosis factor-α and possibly resistin.
- A genetic basis has been confirmed by the identification of variants in the transcription factor-7-like 2 allele and subsequent development of type 2 diabetes.
- The usefulness of the metabolic syndrome as a predictor of diabetes is still debated. β cell dysfunction is present at the diagnosis of type 2 diabetes and gradually declines with time.

Epidemiological studies of diabetes prevalence are often based upon age and self-reported diagnosis. Consequently differentiating type 1 and type 2 patients in population studies is difficult. The most recent authoritative review of global prevalence published by the International Diabetes Federation (IDF) acknowledges these drawbacks. However, as 85–95% globally of all adult diabetes is type 2 then total prevalence rates will overwhelmingly relate to it.

The IDF has also published adult prevalence rates for impaired glucose tolerance (IGT) which closely reflect those for type 2 diabetes. Conversion rates from IGT to diabetes have been reported at 5–11% per annum.

Prevalence

Overall prevalence corrected for age for both type 2 diabetes and IGT is set to increase from 6.0% to 7.3% and 7.5% to 8.0% respectively over the 18 years from 2007 to 2025 – an absolute increase from 246 to 380 and 308 to 418 million persons aged 20–79 years, respectively (Figure 7.1).

The highest rates are currently in the Eastern Mediterranean and Middle East with North and South America close behind.

These reflect the increased life expectancy and overall ageing of the North American population (diabetes is more common in older years). In terms of absolute numbers, the Western Pacific region (particularly China) will have the largest increase of nearly 50%, to 100 million people with diabetes by 2025.

The highest number of people with diabetes is currently in the 40–59-year-old age group, but there will be almost parity with 60–79 year olds by 2025, at 166 and 164 million worldwide respectively.

There is considerable variation within each region, however. For example, in the Western Pacific, the tiny island of Nauru has a comparative prevalence in 2007 of 30.7%, whilst nearby Tonga has less than half that rate at 12.9%, the Philippines 7.6% and China 4.1%.

In the European region, comparative rates range from 1.6% in Iceland to 7.9% in Germany, Austria and Switzerland. The UK rate is 2.9% age adjusted and 4.0% absolute, increasing to 3.5% and 4.6% respectively in 2025 (representing an increase from 1.7 to 2.16 million in absolute numbers).

Urban versus rural

There is a global trend for rates of diabetes to increase in populations as they move from a rural to an urban existence. The reasons are unclear but probably relate to both

Handbook of Diabetes, 4th edition. By © Rudy Bilous & Richard Donnelly. Published 2010 by Blackwell Publishing Ltd.

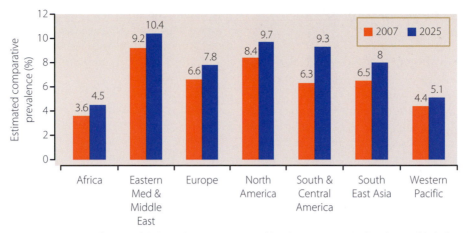

Figure 7.1 Comparative prevalence (corrected for age) of diabetes by region estimated for the years 2007 (red) and 2025 (blue). Data from *Diabetes Atlas*, 3rd edn.

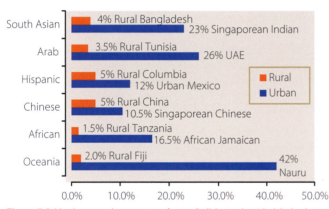

Figure 7.2 Varying prevalence rates of type 2 diabetes by ethnicity/region and location (red, rural; blue, urban) for 2007. UAE, United Arab Emirates. Data from *Diabetes Atlas*, 3rd edn.

decreasing physical activity as well as dietary changes. For example, rural Chinese have a prevalence of type 2 diabetes of 5%, less than half the rate of Singaporean Chinese (10.5%). Much larger differences are seen in South Asian, Hispanic, African and Polynesian peoples (Figure 7.2).

Impaired glucose tolerance

Comparative prevalence for IGT vary by region with rates almost double those for type 2 diabetes in Africa, but slightly lower elsewhere. These differences are almost certainly a reflection of socio-economic factors as well as a paucity of studies in many African countries where extrapolation is necessary between very different populations. In Europe, the comparative prevalence will increase slightly from 9.1% in 2007 to 9.6% in 2025, representing an absolute change from 65.3 to 71.2 million (UK figures 4.7% to 4.9%, 2.17 to 2.4 million respectively).

Incidence

Reported incidence rates vary according to population under study and year of observation. For white Europid populations, rates of 0.1–1% per annum have been reported. For Hispanic populations in the USA, rates of 2.8% were recorded in the San Antonio Study, similar to those of the Pima Indians in Arizona (approximately 2.5%), and Australian aborigines (2.03%).

Over 20 years, incidence in the Pima has not changed although the age of onset has been declining. The occurrence of type 2 diabetes in adolescence is now a great cause for concern worldwide. In US Asian and Pacific Islanders, for example, rates of 12.1/100,000 patient-years have been reported in 10–19 year olds, similar to rates reported for type 1 diabetes. In the UK, the overall incidence for <16 year olds is much lower, at 0.53 per/100,000 patient-years, but 10 times more common in South Asian or black African compared to white children.

The rural:urban ratio remains for incidence even in the presence of other risk factors such as central obesity. In Japanese, there is an approximately threefold increase in incidence for obese urban compared to rural populations (15.8 versus 5.8% over 10 years). Similarly, there is a twofold increase in incidence for USA versus Mexican Hispanic people corrected for age and economic circumstance, probably a reflection of changes in diet and lifestyle. For the Pima, the contrast is more striking, with a >5-fold increase in those living in the US compared to northern Mexico.

The magnitude of these figures has opened a debate on population screening for diabetes, but a Health Technology Assessment report in the UK from 2007 and a report from the US Preventive Services Task Force in 2008 both concluded that there is not enough evidence at present to support such a policy.

Risk factors for development of type 2 diabetes
Obesity

About 80% of people with type 2 diabetes are obese, and the risk of developing diabetes increases progressively as the BMI (weight (kg)/height (m)^2) increases. A BMI >35 kg/m^2 increases the risk of type 2 diabetes developing over a 10-year period by 80-fold, as compared to those with a BMI <22 kg/m^2. Latest data from the NHANES survey in the USA confirm a 6–10-fold increased lifetime risk of type 2 diabetes for 18 year olds with a BMI >35 kg/m^2 compared to those <18.5 kg/m^2 with an associated average 6–7 year reduction in overall life expectancy. Obesity is still widely defined as a BMI >30 kg/m^2 although BMI is not an accurate reflection of fat mass or its distribution, particularly in Asian people. A simple waist circumference may be better (see metabolic syndrome below).

The pattern of obesity is also important in that central fat deposition has a much higher risk for development of diabetes compared to gluteofemoral deposition. In clinical practice such central obesity can be assessed by measuring the weight:hip circumference ratio, but it is unclear whether this has any advantage over a simple waist circumference. Fat deposition at other sites, particularly muscle, liver and islets, may contribute to metabolic defects and insulin resistance (so-called lipotoxicity).

Physical exercise and diet

Low levels of physical exercise also predict the development of type 2 diabetes, possibly because exercise increases insulin sensitivity and helps prevent obesity (Figure 7.4). Subjects who exercise the most have a 25–60% lower risk of developing type 2 diabetes regardless of other risk factors such as obesity and family history.

There has been extensive research into the role of diet as a risk factor for type 2 diabetes. A study in over 10,000 35–55 year olds found that a diet containing large quantities of soft drinks, burgers, sausages and low fibre explained 5.7% of insulin resistance as assessed by the HOMA model. There were 77,440 person-years in the study with 427 incident cases of type 2 diabetes.

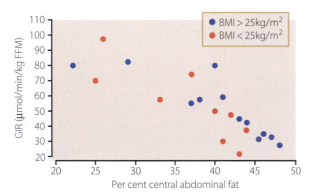

Figure 7.3 Insulin resistance (as assessed by glucose infusion rate (GIR) to maintain constant blood glucose during simultaneous insulin infusion) is proportional to visceral fat mass, independent of BMI. FFM, fat-free mass. Data from Pan et al. Diabetes 1997; 46: 983–988.

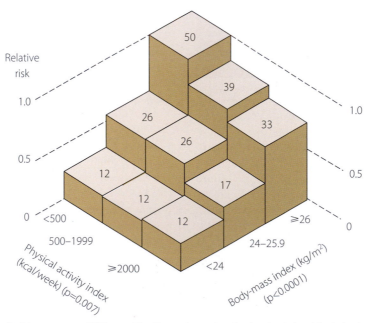

Figure 7.4 Age-adjusted risk of type 2 diabetes among 5990 men. The figure shows data for the physical activity index in relation to BMI. Each block represents the relative risk of type 2 diabetes per 10,000 man-years of follow-up, with the risk for the tallest block set at 1.0. The numbers on the blocks are incidence rates of type 2 diabetes per 10,000 man-years. From Helmrich et al. N Engl J Med 1991; 325: 147–152.

The Diabetes Prevention Programme and Diabetes Prevention Study in the USA and Finland have shown that lifestyle modifications with moderate exercise and modest weight loss can dramatically reduce the number progressing from IGT to type 2 diabetes and reinforce the importance of lifestyle factors in the cause of diabetes.

Insulin resistance

Insulin resistance can be estimated from the amount of glucose that is infused intravenously in order to maintain

a constant blood glucose during a simultaneous intravenous insulin infusion. This method is cumbersome, however, and for population purposes it has been largely superseded by the HOMA (homeostasis model assessment)

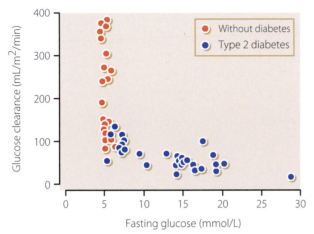

Figure 7.5 The relationship between fasting plasma glucose concentration and glucose metabolic clearance rates (insulin sensitivity) observed during hyperinsulinaemic, glucose-clamp studies in subjects without diabetes and patients with type 2 diabetes. Courtesy of Dr G Reaven, Stanford University School of Medicine, USA.

CASE HISTORY

A 25-year-old single, male postgraduate student, whose parents were from Bangladesh, presented to the local genitourinary clinic with penile candida, and was worried he may have contracted a sexually transmitted disease. Urinalysis confirmed glycosuria and a random capillary blood glucose was 13.2 mmol/L. On direct questioning, he said he had been a bit more thirsty lately. He added that his father had just been diagnosed with type 2 diabetes. He used to play first team hockey as an undergraduate but had stopped following a knee injury 18 months ago. Since then his life had become more sedentary, he ate convenience foods more than four times a week and had gained about 12 kg in weight. He now had a waist circumference of 100 cm and a BMI of 30 kg/m² (weight 86.7 kg, height 1.7 m).

Comment: This young man has multiple risk factors for type 2 diabetes. His ethnic background and family history, recent weight gain, dietary changes and lack of exercise are all well validated. We are not given his birthweight but if this was low then he would also fit the picture of the 'thrifty phenotype'. Although his BMI is definitely raised, his height makes this a less reliable measure of obesity than his waist circumference. He also shows the phenomenon of genetic anticipation in that his age at diagnosis is much earlier than that of his father.

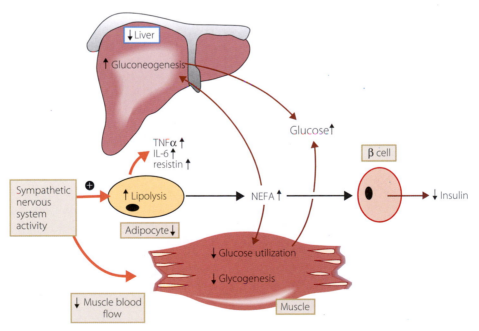

Figure 7.6 Mechanisms of insulin resistance in type 2 diabetes.

estimate of steady-state β cell function (HOMA B) and insulin sensitivity (HOMA S) as percentages of normal. These can be derived from a single fasting plasma C peptide, insulin and glucose concentration. Insulin resistance (or, more correctly, diminished insulin sensitivity) precedes the onset of diabetes and can worsen with increasing duration.

Hormones and cytokines

Visceral fat liberates large amounts of non-esterified fatty acids (NEFAs) through lipolysis, which increases gluconeogenesis in the liver and impairs glucose uptake and utilization in muscle. NEFAs may also inhibit insulin secretion, possibly by enhancing the accumulation of triglyceride within the β cells. In addition, adipose tissue produces cytokines, such as TNF-α, resistin and IL-6, all of which have been shown experimentally to interfere with insulin action. TNF-α has been shown to inhibit tyrosine kinase activity at the insulin receptor and decrease expression of the glucose transporter GLUT-4.

Adiponectin is a hormone with anti-inflammatory and insulin-sensitising properties that is secreted solely by fat cells. It suppresses hepatic gluconeogenesis and stimulates fatty acid oxidation in the liver and skeletal muscles, as well as increasing muscle glucose uptake and insulin release from the β cells. Circulating adiponectin is reduced in obesity and a recent meta-analysis showed that the relative risk for diabetes was 0.72 for every 1-log μg/mL increment in adiponectin level.

Resistin is an adipocyte-secreted hormone that increases insulin resistance and was first described in rodents, being found in increased levels in experimental obesity and diabetes. In humans, it appears to be derived largely from macrophages, however, and its precise role in human diabetes is uncertain, although higher circulating levels have been found in some people with type 2 diabetes.

Leptin is an adipokine that was found to be absent in the ob/ob mouse model of obesity and diabetes. Its normal function is to suppress appetite, thus providing a candidate mechanism linking weight gain and appetite control. Although abnormal leptin function has been described in humans, these defects are very rare and paradoxically high levels have been found in type 2 diabetes.

Ghrelin is a recently described peptide secreted from the stomach and may act as a hunger signal. Circulating levels are negatively correlated with BMI and are suppressed by food intake. It has no known role in human diabetes but antagonism may provide a therapeutic target.

Finally there is often increased sympathetic nervous system activity in obesity, which might also increase lipolysis, reduce muscle blood flow and thus glucose delivery and uptake, and therefore directly affect insulin action.

Inflammation

Many of these cytokines are involved in the acute-phase response and it is therefore not surprising that circulating markers such as C-reactive protein and sialic acid are increased in type 2 diabetic patients, as well as in those who later go on to develop the condition. Because these markers have also been found to be elevated in patients with atherosclerosis, a unifying hypothesis has evolved proposing that inflammation may be a common precursor and link between diabetes and coronary artery disease.

Genetics

Evidence for a genetic basis for type 2 diabetes comes from a clear familial aggregation, but it does not segregate in a classic Mendelian fashion. About 10% of patients with type 2 diabetes have a similarly affected sibling. The concordance rate for identical twins is variously estimated to be 33–90% (17–37% in non-identical twins), but the interpretation of this is controversial as part of the explanation for the high concordance may be environmental rather than genetic.

Unlike type 1, type 2 diabetes is not associated with genes in the HLA region. So far, 19 gene variants have been described and validated as being associated with type 2 diabetes. Of these, the strongest is TCF7L2; 15% of European adults carry two copies of the abnormal gene and they have double the lifetime risk of developing type 2 diabetes compared to the 40% who carry no copies. Carriers of the T risk allele have impaired insulin secretion and enhanced hepatic glucose output. Nearly all of the other described genes affect either β cell mass or function; few appear to have potential effects on insulin resistance.

Thrifty phenotype hypothesis

A link between low birthweight and later development of type 2 diabetes in a UK population has led to a hypothesis linking foetal malnutrition to impaired β cell development and insulin resistance in adulthood. Abundant adult nutrition and consequent obesity would then expose these problems, leading to IGT and eventually type 2 diabetes. This has been called the thrifty phenotype hypothesis (Figure 7.7).

A meta-analysis of 31 populations involving 152,084 individuals from varying ethnic groups and 6090 cases of diabetes was published in 2008. This confirmed a negative association between birthweight and diabetes in 23, but found a positive association in eight studies. The combined odds ratio for type 2 diabetes was 0.8 (95% CI 0.72–0.89) for each 1 kg increase in birthweight. This relationship was strengthened if macrosomic (birthweight >4 kg) and offspring of mothers with known type 2 diabetes were excluded (odds ratio (OR) 0.67, 95% CI 0.61–0.73). Notably there was a tendency for a positive relationship in North American populations largely due to higher rates of maternal obesity and gestational diabetes. Adjustment for socio-economic

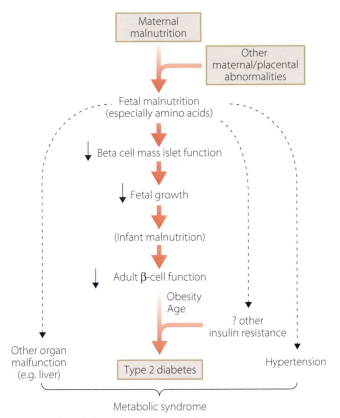

Figure 7.7 The 'thrifty phenotype' hypothesis.

Table 7.1 Definition of metabolic syndrome

Risk factor	Defining level	
	NCEP ATP III	IDF
Abdominal obesity (waist circumference)		
Men	>102 cm	≥94 cm (Europid) ≥90 cm (others)
Women	>88 cm	≥80 cm for all
Plasma triglycerides	≥1.7 mmol/L	≥1.7 mmol/L
Plasma HDL cholesterol		
Men	<0.9 mmol/L	<1.03 mmol/L
Women	<1.1 mmol/L	<1.29 mmol/L
Blood pressure	≥130/≥85 mmHg	≥130/≥85 mmHg or on treatment
Plasma fasting glucose	≥6.1 mmol/L	≥5.6 mmol/L or pre-existing type 2 diabetes
Diagnostic criteria	3 or more of the above	Obesity plus 2 others

NCEP ATP III, National Cholesterol Education Programme – 3rd Adult Treatment Panel; IDF, International Diabetes Federation.

status had no effect, but adjustment for achieved adult BMI attenuated the relationship.

With increasing maternal obesity and gestational diabetes mellitus (GDM), it is conceivable that the relationship will change to the pattern currently seen in Native Americans which is more U shaped. However, it is still unclear whether low birthweight is a causative factor or a sign of other potential mechanisms which may predispose to later diabetes.

Accelerator hypothesis

This is a proposal that type 1 and type 2 diabetes are essentially the same in that both result ultimately from β cell failure. The aetiology obviously differs but superimposed insulin resistance drives the process. Three accelerators are proposed: constitution – individuals have increased β cell apoptosis; insulin resistance – underpinned by physical inactivity and visceral adiposity; and autoimmunity – mainly operative in younger patients and linked to HLA susceptibility alleles. The overlapping driver of obesity would explain increasing rates of 'type 1' and 'type 2' diabetes. This intriguing idea is currently widely debated and awaits confirmatory studies.

Metabolic syndrome

The aggregation of obesity, hyperglycaemia, hypertension and hyperlipidaemia in people with both type 2 diabetes and cardiovascular disease is now termed the metabolic syndrome (Table 7.1). This concept is not new, it is said to have been first described in 1923, but latterly there have been attempts to standardise its definition.

Since these definitions appeared, there has been considerable debate as to their relative strengths and weaknesses. Indeed, there is some debate as to whether this constitutes a true syndrome at all and whether they add anything to predictive models for type 2 diabetes and coronary artery disease. A major problem is the correlation of many of the features. In prospective studies, fasting plasma glucose (FPG) is overwhelmingly linked to subsequent development of diabetes, but much less so with coronary artery disease. Thus the predictive utility of the metabolic syndrome as a concept adds little to its constituent risk factors when they are used individually. The long-term usefulness of the definition of the metabolic syndrome for identification and intervention in order to prevent diabetes and cardiovascular disease has yet to be demonstrated.

β cell dysfunction

Type 2 diabetes develops because of a progressive deterioration of β cell function, coupled with increasing insulin resistance for which the β cell cannot compensate. At the time of diagnosis β cell function is already reduced by about 50% and continues to decline regardless of therapy (Figure 7.8).

The main defects in β cell function in type 2 diabetes are a markedly reduced first- and second-phase insulin response to intravenous glucose, and a delayed or blunted response

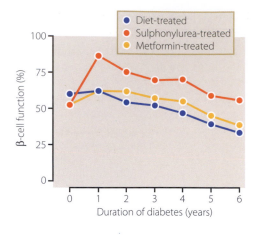

Figure 7.8 β-cell function as measured by the homeostasis model assessment (HOMA) method (calculated from the fasting blood glucose and insulin concentrations) in patients with type 2 diabetes from the UKPDS. β cell function is already reduced to 50% at diagnosis and declines thereafter, despite therapy. Data from Hales & Barker. Diabetologia 1992; 35: 595–601.

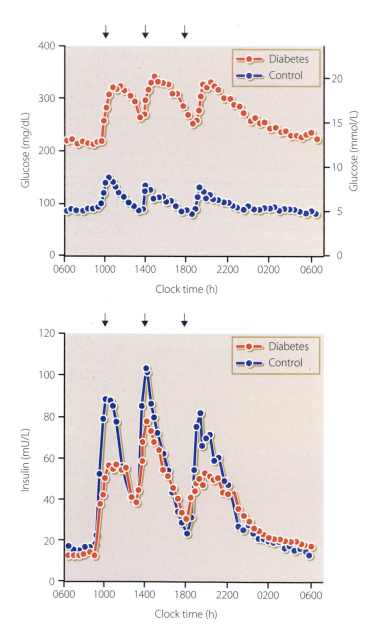

Figure 7.9 Plasma concentrations of glucose and insulin in subjects with type 2 diabetes and control subjects without diabetes in response to mixed meals. Data from UK Prospective Diabetes Study Group. Diabetes 1995; 44:1249–1258.

to mixed meals (Figure 7.9). There are also alterations in pulsatile and daytime oscillations of insulin release. Some researchers have found increases in the proportions of plasma proinsulin and split proinsulin peptides relative to insulin alone. Many of these abnormalities can be found in people with IGT and even in normoglycaemic first-degree relatives of people with type 2 diabetes, indicating that impaired β cell function is an early and possibly genetic defect in the natural history of type 2 diabetes (Figure 7.10).

The most common histological abnormality found in the islets of patients with type 2 diabetes is the presence of insoluble amyloid fibrils lying outside the cells. These are derived from islet amyloid polypeptide (IAPP, also sometimes known as amylin). This is co-secreted with insulin in a molar ratio of 1:10–50. Although IAPP is reported to impair insulin secretion and to be toxic to the β cell, its precise role in the pathogenesis of type 2 diabetes is uncertain because deposits can be found in up to 20% of elderly people who had completely normal glucose tolerance in life.

β Cell mass is thought to be decreased by only 20–40% in type 2 diabetes and this clearly cannot explain the >80% reduction in insulin release that is observed. There must therefore be additional functional defects in the β cell, perhaps mediated by glucose or lipid toxicity. It is likely that IAPP contributes to this process.

Conclusion

Both insulin resistance and β cell dysfunction are early features of glucose intolerance, and there has been much debate as to whether one is the primary defect and precedes the other. In practice, the contribution of insulin resistance and β cell dysfunction varies considerably between patients,

LANDMARK CLINICAL TRIALS

Diabetes Prevention Program Research Group. Reduction in incidence of type 2 diabetes with lifestyle intervention or metformin. N Engl J Med 2002; 346: 393–403.

Lindstrom J, Ilanne-Parikka P, Peltonen M, et al. Sustained reduction in the incidence of type 2 diabetes by lifestyle intervention: follow-up of the Finnish Diabetes Prevention Study. Lancet 2006; 368: 1673–1679.

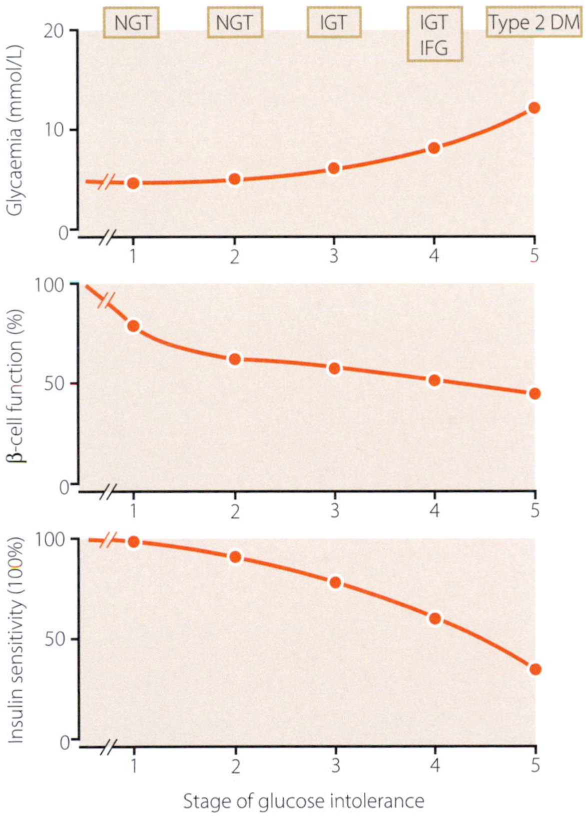

Figure 7.10 The stages of glucose tolerance and associated β cell function and insulin sensitivity, from normal glucose tolerance (NGT) through impaired glucose tolerance (IGT), with or without impaired fasting glucose (IFG), and finally type 2 diabetes mellitus (DM). Courtesy of Dr H Lewis Jones, Liverpool University, UK.

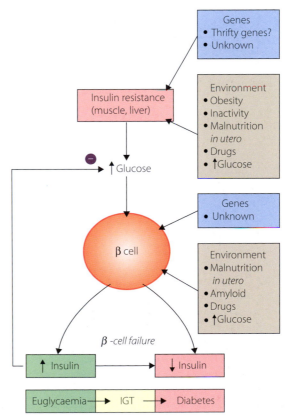

Figure 7.11 Pathogenesis of type 2 diabetes. Both genetic and environmental factors contribute to both insulin resistance and β cell failure.

as well as during the course of the disease. Usually, there is a decline in both insulin sensitivity and insulin secretion in patients who progress from IGT to diabetes and undoubtedly environmental and genetic factors contribute to this process (Figure 7.11).

KEY WEBSITES

- Diabetes atlas for prevalence/incidence: www.eatlas.idf.org
- HOMA calculator: www.dtu.ox.ac.uk

FURTHER READING

Alberti KG, Zimmet P, Shaw J. Metabolic syndrome – a new worldwide definition. A consensus statement from the International Diabetes Federation. Diabetic Med 2006; 23: 469–480.

Expert Panel On Detection, Evaluation And Treatment Of High Blood Cholesterol In Adults (Adult Treatment Panel III). Executive summary of the 3rd report of the National Cholesterol Education Programme (NCEP). JAMA 2001; 285: 2486–2497.

International Diabetes Federation. *Diabetes Atlas*, 4th edn. Brussels: International Diabetes Federation, 2009.

Kahn R, Buse J, Ferrannini E, Stern M. The metabolic syndrome: time for a critical appraisal. Joint statement from the American Diabetes Association and the European Association for the Study of Diabetes. Diabetes Care 2005; 28: 2289–2304.

Li S, Shin HJ, Ding EL, van Dam RM. Adiponectin levels and risk of type 2 diabetes. A systematic review and meta-analysis. JAMA 2009; 302: 179–188.

Maleciki MT. Genetics of type 2 diabetes mellitus. Diabet Res Clin Pract 2005; 68(Suppl 1): S10–S21.

Nomi SL, Kansagara D, Bougatsos C, Fu R, US Preventive Services Task Force. Screening adults for type 2 diabetes: a review of the evidence for the US Preventive Services Task Force. Ann Intern Med 2008; 148: 855–868.

Sparso T, Grarup N, Andreasen C, et al. Combined analysis of 19 common validated type 2 diabetes susceptibility gene variants shows moderate discriminative value and no evidence of gene-gene interaction. Diabetologia 2009; 52: 1308–1314.

Waugh N, Scotland G, McName P, et al. Screening for type 2 diabetes: literature review and economic modelling. Health Technol Assess 2007; 11: 1–125.

Whincup PH, Kaye SJ, Owen CG, et al. Birth weight and risk of type 2 diabetes mellitus. JAMA 2008; 300: 2886–2897.

Other types of diabetes

Maturity-onset diabetes of the young

Maturity-onset diabetes of the young (MODY) owes its name to a time when diabetes was defined by age of onset. The nomenclature has stuck, however, and MODY defines usually non-insulin dependent diabetes occurring before the age of 25 years and with a striking autosomal dominant inheritance. β cell dysfunction is usually present but in contrast to type 2 diabetes, obesity and insulin resistance are unusual. MODY accounts for about 1–2% of patients with diabetes in most white Europid populations. The diagnostic criteria which should suggest a diagnosis of MODY are listed in Box 8.1.

A recent survey of newly presenting non-type 1 diabetes in children <16 years of age in the UK revealed 17 cases of MODY, giving an incidence of 0.13/100,000 patient-years. This is almost certainly an underestimate as MODY 2 is often undetected for many years because it is largely asymptomatic.

The most common causes (accounting for >75% of cases) are mutations in nuclear transcription factors that control insulin production and secretion. They are listed in Table 8.1 together with associated clinical features. MODY 2 is a defect in the glucose-sensing glucokinase enzyme which means that insulin release occurs at higher than usual circulating blood glucose levels, usually leading to a raised fasting blood

Handbook of Diabetes, 4th edition. By © Rudy Bilous & Richard Donnelly. Published 2010 by Blackwell Publishing Ltd.

Box 8.1 Diagnostic criteria for MODY

- Early diagnosis of diabetes – usually before age 25 years in at least one family member
- Non-insulin requiring – shown by absence of insulin treatment 5 years after diagnosis or the demonstration of significant circulating C-peptide in a patient on insulin treatment
- Autosomal-dominant inheritance with vertical transmission through at least two generations (ideally three), with a similar phenotype in affected individuals

glucose. These patients are commonly detected either in pregnancy during screening for gestational diabetes, or as part of a health screening programme. MODY 2 needs no treatment, is largely benign and not associated with diabetes complications.

Other forms of MODY, however, are progressive and require treatment. Sulphonylureas are often initially effective but many patients ultimately need insulin. Because blood glucose levels are higher than MODY 2, these patients are prone to both micro- and macrovascular complications.

Pancreatic disease

Many pancreatic diseases can cause diabetes, but in total they account for <1% of all cases. Acute pancreatitis (commonly associated with alcoholism or gallstones) (Figure 8.1)

Table 8.1 Different genetic aetiologies of MODY

Genetic basis	Clinical and biochemical features	Frequency
HNF4α (MODY1)	Low fasting triglycerides. Increased birthweight. Reduced apolipoproteins apo A11 and apo C111. Responds to sulphonylureas	3%
Glucokinase (MODY 2)	β cell response to high blood glucose impaired. Mild fasting hyperglycaemia, can present as gestational diabetes. Usually does not require treatment	14%
HNF1α (MODY 3)	Raised HDL cholesterol. Responds well to sulphonylureas	69%
IPF-1 (MODY 4)	Pancreatic agenesis with homozygous mutations	<1%
HNF1-β (MODY 5)	Renal abnormalities (cysts, dysplasia). Uterine and genital abnormalities. Short stature and low birthweight. Pancreatic atrophy	3%
NEURO D1 (MODY 6)	None described but probably reduced β cell formation	<1%
KLF 11 (MODY 7)	None described	<1%
CEL (MODY 8)	Pancreatic atrophy with exocrine deficiency	<1%
MODY X	Unknown and gene defect yet to be determined	10%

HNF, hepatocyte nuclear factor; IPF, insulin promotor factor; NEURO D1, neurogenic differentiating factor 1; KLF, Kruppel-like factor; CEL, carboxyl-ester-lipase.

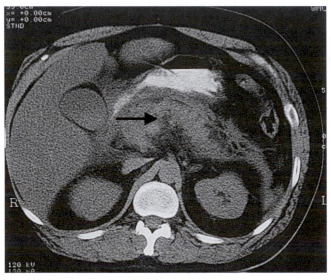

Figure 8.1 Acute pancreatitis. CT scan of the abdomen, showing marked oedema and swelling of the gland (arrow). Subsequently, a pancreatic pseudocyst developed.

usually results in transient hyperglycaemia, but permanent diabetes occurs in up to 15% of patients.

Chronic pancreatitis, which is commonly caused by alcoholism in Western countries, leads to IGT or diabetes in 40–50% of cases. Intraductal protein plugs subsequently calcify as characteristic calcite stones, with cyst formation, inflammation and fibrosis. One-third require insulin, but ketoacidosis is rare. Many patients are extremely insulin sensitive, requiring small doses to prevent ketosis; higher doses are often associated with hypoglycaemia.

Tropical calcific pancreatitis is confined to India and developing nations, and results in diabetes in 90% of cases. Even in these countries, it accounts for only 1% of diabetes.

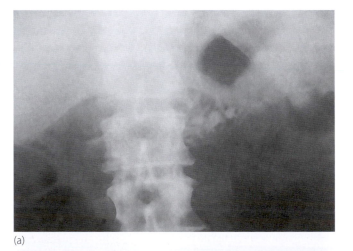

(a)

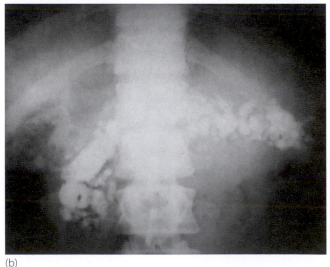

(b)

Figure 8.2 Pancreatic calculi, showing characteristic patterns in alcoholic chronic pancreatitis (a), and fibrocalculous pancreatic diabetes (b).

It is often associated with malnutrition, its aetiology is not understood and most patients require insulin.

Cystic fibrosis

This is a common autosomal recessive condition which results in abnormal chloride and water transport across epithelial membranes. Over 1500 mutations in the cystic fibrosis transmembrane conductance regulator gene have been described and they result in differing severities of the condition. Pancreatic and pulmonary disease predominate and better treatment has resulted in much improved survival. Diabetes results from β cell failure secondary to exocrine pancreatic damage. A recent UK survey of 8029 patients on the cystic fibrosis register studied from 1996 to 2005 revealed an annual incidence of diabetes of 3.5%, but this was 1–2% in the first decade of life, and 6–7% in the fourth. Female sex, more severe lung dysfunction, liver disease, exocrine pancreatic insufficiency, steroid use and severity of gene expression were all positively related to diabetes development.

The earliest biochemical abnormality tends to be postprandial hyperglycaemia. The majority of patients require insulin treatment.

Haemochromatosis

This is an autosomal recessive inborn error of metabolism, usually caused by a mutation in the haemochromatosis gene, HFE, on chromosome 6. The HFE protein is expressed on duodenal enterocytes and modulates iron uptake. Haemochromatosis is associated with increased iron absorption and tissue deposition, notably in the liver, pancreatic islets, skin and pituitary glands. The classic clinical triad is one of hepatic cirrhosis, glucose intolerance with insulin-requiring diabetes in 25%, and skin hyperpigmentation, which has led to the term 'bronzed diabetes'. Serum iron and ferritin concentrations are raised. Secondary haemochromatosis may occur in patients who undergo frequent blood transfusions, for example those with β-thalassaemia or other haemoglobinopathies.

Pancreatic cancer

Rarely, diabetes can be a presenting feature of pancreatic cancer. Usually, however, there are other features such as profound weight loss and back pain. The prognosis is very poor; insulin treatment is usual.

Neonatal diabetes

Permanent neonatal diabetes (PNDM) is caused by a mutation in the gene coding the Kir 6.2 and SUR1 sub units of the KATP channel on the β cell. This defect results in an inability to release insulin and consequent ketoacidosis, usually occurring before 6 months of age. Sulphonylureas close this channel by an ATP-independent route and are effective in over 50% of cases of PNDM.

Mitochrondrial diabetes

Mitochrondrial DNA is inherited maternally. A heteroplasmic mutation at position 3243 results in type 2 diabetes and sensorineural deafness. Other features include myopathy, pigmented retinopathy, cardiomyopathy and neurological abnormalities. Its most severe form comprises the MELAS syndrome (Myopathy, Encephalopathy, Lactic Acidosis and Stroke-like episodes). Prevalence studies suggest that Mt 3243 accounts for 1–2% of Japanese and 0.2–0.5% of European type 2 diabetes.

Wolfram syndrome

This rare autosomal recessive disorder was first described in 1938. The most common features are Diabetes Insipidus, type 1 Diabetes Mellitus, Optic Atrophy (Figure 8.3) and Deafness (DIDMOAD). There are many other features, notably psychiatric illness. A gene defect on chromosome 4 coding for a transmembrane protein (wolframmin) has been described, together with some mitochondrial DNA abnormalities (but not 3243). Diabetes usually occurs in the second decade and prevalence has been estimated as between 1 in 100,000 – 800,000 of the population.

Lipodystrophies

These are rare inherited conditions characterised by a partial or total absence of adipose tissue and have an associated

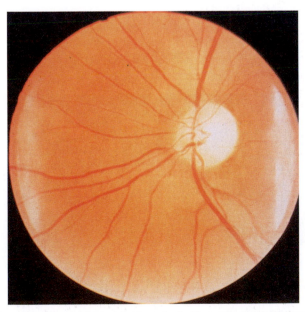

Figure 8.3 Optic atrophy (note white optic disc) in a patient with Wolfram's syndrome.

insulin resistance. In many cases, the genetic basis has been discovered, leading to new insights into the causes of insulin resistance. Patients with partial lipodystrophy (sometimes called the Kobberling–Dunnigan syndrome) have an abnormality in the LMNA (encoding lamin A/C which is a constituent of nuclear lamina) or PPAR γ gene. These changes result in defective adipocyte differentiation and/or cell death. Apart from type 2 diabetes, some of these patients also have problems with severe hypertriglyceridaemia, hepatic steatosis and pancreatitis.

Generalised lipoatrophy usually presents in early childhood and several different genetic causes have been described for this. Severe insulin resistance, diabetes and hyperlipidaemia are the norm.

Myotonic dystrophy

This autosomal dominant disorder is the most common adult form of muscular dystrophy (prevalence 1 in 8000 population) and is characterised by abnormal insulin secretion, insulin resistance and type 2 diabetes. The abnormal mutation is in the protein kinase gene on chromosome 19 and this may affect insulin receptor RNA and protein expression or perhaps calcium-dependent insulin release from the β cells.

Abnormalities of the insulin receptor or insulin molecule

Genetic abnormalities in the insulin receptor can give rise to rare but well-described syndromes characterised by severe insulin resistance. Clinically these patients have acanthosis nigricans (hyperpigmented velvety skin in the flexures of the neck, axillae or groin) (Figure 8.4) and hyperandrogenism.

Mutations of the gene encoding the α subunit of the insulin receptor can lead to leprechaunism or the less severe Rabson–Mendenhall syndrome (Figure 8.5).

CASE HISTORY

A 22-year-old woman was referred to the medical obstetrics clinic for booking at 6 weeks gestation of her first pregnancy. She had had diabetes for 10 years, initially on sulphonylureas for 6 months but now on insulin. She had never been ketotic. Her control was fair (HbA$_{1c}$ 8.2%). She had a strong family history of diabetes; her mother had type 2 diabetes and was now on insulin and currently an inpatient, having required a below-knee amputation for neuroischaemia and gangrene. Her brother was in the army and had recently been diagnosed with type 2 diabetes at the age of 19 years. Another brother aged 24 years had had diet-controlled diabetes for 6 years.

DNA testing revealed a mutation in the HNF1α gene, confirming a diagnosis of MODY 3. During pregnancy her glycaemic control improved dramatically but unfortunately she developed rapidly progressive retinopathy requiring laser photocoagulation. Postpartum she was tried again on sulphonylureas but her glycaemia worsened and she was recommenced on insulin. Three years later she has established nephropathy and has required vitreoretinal surgery.

Comment: This case shows many of the typical features of MODY as outlined in Box 8.1. Not all can be managed on oral agents and many are prone to severe complications. This woman and her family have received counselling from the UK Regional MODY Service.

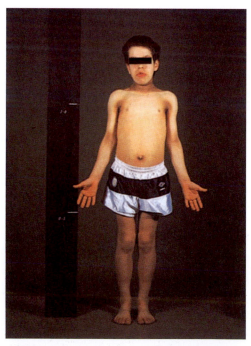

Figure 8.5 Rabson–Mendenhall syndrome in a 12-year-old boy, showing growth retardation, prominent acanthosis nigricans affecting the axillae, neck and antecubital fossae, and typical facies.

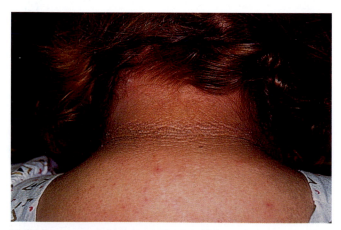

Figure 8.4 Acanthosis nigricans on the nape of the neck of a 26-year-old woman with the type A insulin resistance syndrome.

Type A insulin resistance affects mainly adolescent girls and shares many features with the polycystic ovary syndrome (Figure 8.4). In 25% of cases there is a mutation of the tyrosine kinase domain of the β subunit of the insulin receptor.

Rare mutations of the human preproinsulin gene can lead to abnormal levels of insulin precursors. Such patients are heterozygous (homozygosity would be incompatible with life), and develop diabetes in later life in response to other factors such as obesity.

Autoimmune insulin resistance

Type B insulin resistance is very rare and the result of circulating antibodies to the insulin receptor. There is a link with other autoimmune diseases and with these shares a female preponderance. Patients may have fluctuating hyper- and hypoglycaemia and are very difficult to treat.

Diabetes complicating other endocrine diseases

Several endocrine conditions are associated with diabetes mellitus. Cushing's syndrome is the result of glucocorticoid excess from any cause, including steroid drug induced, pituitary adenomas, adrenal tumours and ectopic ACTH production. Glucocorticoid excess results in central obesity which causes insulin resistance. This in turn stimulates hepatic gluconeogenesis, peripheral adipose tissue lipolysis and NEFA release. All of these inhibit peripheral glucose uptake and the net result is hyperglycaemia. Most patients have some degree of glucose intolerance, with overt diabetes in 10–20% of cases.

Acromegaly is a condition of growth hormone excess almost always arising from an anterior pituitary tumour. This causes glucose intolerance by inducing insulin resistance. Overt diabetes and impaired glucose tolerance each affect around one-third of patients with acromegaly. Glucose tolerance returns to normal with effective treatment and reduction of circulating growth hormone levels.

Phaeochromocytomas are tumours that arise from the chromaffin cells of the sympathetic nervous system, usually in the adrenal medulla but they can occur anywhere along the sympathetic nervous chain. They secrete excess catecholamines, and typically the clinical presentation is that of high blood pressure, headache, tachycardia and sweating, sometimes occurring in paroxysms. Up to 75% have evidence of glucose intolerance but this rarely needs treatment with insulin. Resolution is usual with removal of the tumour.

Glucagonomas are rare tumours of the islet α cells (Figure 8.6). They are slowly growing but often malignant. The most striking clinical features are weight loss and a characteristic rash, termed 'necrolytic migratory erythema' affecting skin flexures and the perineum. There is also a tendency to

thromboembolism and neuropsychiatric disorders. Diabetes is common and the result of enhanced gluconeogenesis and glycogenolysis induced by high circulating glucagon levels. It usually resolves with removal of the tumour.

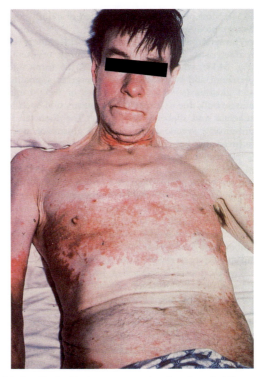

Figure 8.6 A patient with glucagonoma, showing characteristic necrolytic migratory erythema. Non-ketotic diabetes was controlled with low doses of insulin.

KEY WEBSITES

- Diagnostic criteria and details of how to request genetic tests for MODY in the UK: http://projects.exeter.ac.uk/diabetesgenes/mody/
- Information on monogeneic form of diabetes: http://diabetes.niddk.nih.gov/dm/pubs/mody/

FURTHER READING

Adler AI, Shine BSF, Chamnan P, Haworth CS, Bilton D. Genetic determinance and epidemiology of cystic fibrosis-related diabetes: results from a British cohort of children and adults. Diabetes Care 2008; 31: 1789–1794.

American Diabetes Association. Diagnosis and classification of diabetes mellitus. Diabetes Care 2010; 33(Suppl 1): S62–S69.

Garg A. Acquired and inherited lipodystrophies. N Engl J Med 2004; 350: 1220–1234.

Maleciki MT. Genetics of type 2 diabetes mellitus. Diabet Res Clin Pract 2005; 68(Suppl 1): S10–S21.

McCarthy MI, Hattersley AT. Learning from molecular genetics. Diabetes 2008; 57: 2889–2898.

Part 2

Metabolic control and complications

Diabetes control and its measurement

'Diabetic control' defines the extent to which the metabolism in the person with diabetes differs from that in the person without diabetes. Measurement usually focuses on blood glucose: 'good' control implies maintenance of near-normal blood glucose concentrations throughout the day. However, many other metabolites are disordered in diabetes and some, such as ketone bodies, are now more easily measurable and clinically useful, particularly during acute illness or periods of poor blood glucose control (Figure 9.1).

In addition to blood and urine glucose concentrations, there are indicators of longer term glycaemic control over the preceding weeks using plasma glycated haemoglobin (HbA_{1c}) or fructosamine concentrations (Table 9.1).

Capillary blood glucose monitoring

Single blood glucose measurements are of little use as an assessment of overall control in type 1 diabetes because of unpredictable variations throughout the day and from day to day, although they are important in order to detect hypoglycaemia. In order to assess control more meaningfully, serial, timed blood glucose samples are usually needed. In diet- or stable tablet-controlled type 2 diabetes, although blood glucose levels are elevated they tend not to vary widely throughout the day. In these patients a fasting or random blood glucose relates reasonably well to mean blood glucose concentration and to glycated haemoglobin and is probably adequate.

Self-monitoring of capillary blood glucose by patients at home using special enzyme-impregnated reagent strips and a meter is now an integral part of modern diabetes management, especially for those who are on insulin therapy (Figure 9.2). Strips usually contain a combination of glucose oxidase and peroxidase. Colorimetric tests have now largely been superceded by newer electrochemically based strips which generate a current rather than a colour change. Meters vary in their need for standardisation, their memory and their ability to generate blood glucose profiles when connected to a computer. Some contain algorithms that can give advice on insulin dosage prior to a meal, depending on its carbohydrate content. Some meters require more blood than others. Meters are often made freely available by the manufacturers in the UK.

It is worth remembering that all meters tend to be less accurate at lower blood glucose values and usually have an upper limit of detection following which they read 'high'.

There are many devices which contain a spring-loaded lancet in order to obtain a capillary blood sample (Figure 9.2). This is usually obtained from the fingers; the sides of the fingertip are less sensitive than the pulp. A major reason for poor compliance and low frequency of testing is finger

Handbook of Diabetes, 4th edition. By © Rudy Bilous & Richard Donnelly. Published 2010 by Blackwell Publishing Ltd.

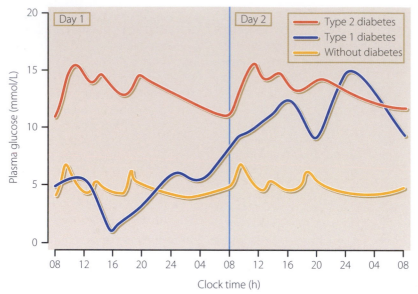

Figure 9.1 Variations in plasma glucose concentrations over 2 days in a person without diabetes, a patient with type 1 diabetes (wide swings in glucose levels with little day-to-day consistency) and a patient with type 2 diabetes (similar profile to a subject without diabetes, but at a higher level and with greater postprandial peaks; fairly consistent from day to day). From Pickup & Williams. *Textbook of Diabetes*, 3rd edition. Blackwell Publishing Ltd, 2003.

Table 9.1 Indicators of glycaemic control

Indicator	Main clinical use
Urine glucose	Poor index of BG, useful for surveillance in stable non-insulin treated type 2 diabetes
Blood glucose	
• Fasting	Correlates with mean daily BG and HbA$_{1c}$ in type 2 diabetes
• Diurnal/circadian profiles	Self-monitoring of BG, hospital assessment
Glycated haemoglobin	Glycaemic control (mean) over preceding 1–3 months
Glycated serum protein, e.g. fructosamine	Glycaemic control (mean) over preceding 2 weeks
Urine and blood ketones	Insulin deficiency, warning of DKA, monitoring during intercurrent illness
Other blood metabolites/ hormones	
• Cholesterol (total and HDL) and triglyceride	Cardiovascular risk factors

BG, blood glucose; DKA, diabetic ketoacidosis; HbA$_{1c}$, glycated haemoglobin.

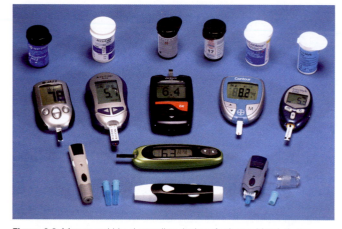

Figure 9.2 Meters and blood sampling devices for home blood glucose monitoring.

discomfort. In recent years strips require less blood and many devices have a depth adjustment. Some offer the option of testing at alternative sites to the fingers such as the forearm, abdomen, calf and thigh. However, there can be discrepancies in values measured at the finger and these sites, particularly during times of rapid change in blood glucose such as after meals or exercise.

Frequency of testing

Initial trials of home blood glucose monitoring were nothing short of revelatory for patients used to urine tests. Latterly, as part of clinical trials (e.g. Diabetes Control and Complications Trial (DCCT) in type 1 and UK Prospective Diabetes Study (UKPDS) in type 2) and structured educational programmes (e.g. Diet Adjustment For Normal Eating (DAFNE) in the UK), they have been shown to help patients achieve sustained long-term improvements in glycaemic control. However, systematic reviews have failed to confirm that home blood glucose monitoring alone results in significant glycaemic improvement. Many patients, though, prefer it to urinalysis, and it is hard to see how multiple daily insulin injection regimens can be used without it. NICE guidance uses it as an essential component of care management in type 1 diabetes with a frequency dependent upon the clinical circumstances, whereas for type 2 diabetes home blood glucose monitoring should be available for the indications listed in Box 9.1. Both NICE type 1 and type 2 guidelines suggest that knowledge and skills of interpretation, and action based upon home blood glucose monitoring results should be assessed annually. The American Diabetes Association guidelines suggest three or more tests per day in type 1 diabetes on multiple daily injections or pump therapy and for pregnant women. Otherwise their advice is concordant with that from NICE.

Urine glucose monitoring

Glycosuria occurs when blood glucose levels exceed the renal threshold for glucose (usually 10 mmol/L–180 mg/dL). However, urine glucose testing is unreliable in the assessment of blood glucose control because renal threshold varies between and within patients (Box 9.2). Fluid intake can affect urine glucose concentrations and importantly, the result does not reflect blood glucose at the time of the test but over the duration that the urine has accumulated in the bladder. A negative urine test cannot distinguish between hypoglycaemia, normoglycaemia and modest hyperglycaemia.

However, urine testing still remains a reasonable option in stable type 2 diabetic patients treated with diet or oral agents, particularly in those who are unable or unwilling to perform blood glucose monitoring. It should be supplemented by glycated haemoglobin tests once or twice a year. It is worth noting that there is no benefit in terms of assessment of control in using freshly voided urine samples.

Box 9.1 Indications for capillary blood glucose monitoring in type 2 diabetes

- Insulin therapy
- On oral therapy with a risk of hypoglycaemia (e.g. sulphonylureas, glitinides)
- Assessment of response of glycaemia to changes in management or lifestyle
- Monitoring of glycaemia during intercurrent illness
- Avoidance of hypoglycaemia during driving, employment or physical activity

---

Box 9.2 Limitations of urine testing for glucose

- Variations in renal threshold, especially in pregnancy
- Variable result depending on urinary output/concentration
- No immediate relationship to current blood glucose
- Negative test unhelpful for detection of hypoglycaemia
- Visual reading of colour required
- Accuracy may not be as precise at urine concentrations around 5.5 mmol/L
- Some drugs may interfere with the test

Glycated haemoglobin

Haemoglobin A comprises over 90% of most adult haemoglobin and is variably glycated by the non-enzymatic attachment of sugars. HbA_{1c} comprises the major glycated component and has been shown in numerous studies to correlate with average blood glucose (Figure 9.3).

As the average life span of the red cell is 90–120 days, the percentage glycated haemoglobin is a reflection of glycaemic control over the 8–12 weeks preceding the test. However, the level of glycation is not linear with time – 50% of the value reflects the 30 days prior to the test, and only 10% the initial 30 days of red cell life.

It is important to remember this because if the life span of a patient's red cell is less than 90 days then theoretically the HbA_{1c} could be 50% of the expected value. Although high-pressure liquid chromatography (HPLC) methodology and the new International Federation for Clinical Chemistry and Laboratory Medicine (IFCC) standard have largely eliminated the confounding problems of aberrant haemoglobins, these can still cause falsely high values in some populations where they exist in high prevalence. It is important to check local assays in order to be aware of potential confounding factors.

The more common causes of misleading HbA_{1c} values are shown in Box 9.3. Carbamylation due to uraemia increases HbA_{1c} by 0.063% for every 1 mmol/L increase in plasma urea concentration so is of relatively minor consequence.

Of more importance is the observation that there is considerable interindividual variation in the correlation between average blood glucose and HbA_{1c}. Analysis of the DCCT

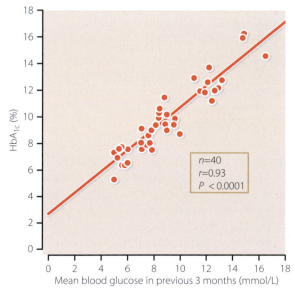

Figure 9.3 Correlation in patients with type 1 diabetes between blood glucose concentration over the preceding 3 months and glycated haemoglobin (HbA_{1c}) level. Adapted from Paisey. Diabetologia 1980; 19: 31–34.

Box 9.3 Potential reasons for a misleading HbA$_{1c}$

Altered red blood cell turnover
- Blood loss
- Haemolysis
- Haemoglobinopathies and red cell disorders
- Myelodysplasia
- Pregnancy
- Iron deficiency

Interference with assay
- Persistent foetal haemoglobin
- Haemoglobin variant
- Carbamylation

Timing
- Too frequent testing

Imprecision
- Differences of approximately 0.4% reflect ± 2 SD for most modern assays

Variability in red blood cell membrane transport (slow/rapid glycators)

Table 9.2 Correlation of HbA$_{1c}$ with average blood glucose (r = 0.92) (based upon ADAG Trial)

HbA$_{1c}$ %	Mean blood glucose	
	mmol/L	mg/dL
6	7.0	126
7	8.6	154
8	10.2	183
9	11.8	212
10	13.4	240
11	14.9	269
12	16.5	298

(r = 0.92) has not been reproduced in children and there may also be differences in African Americans. There is ongoing debate about the utility of eAG and there are as yet no data to suggest it has clinical benefit over and above HbA$_{1c}$. It is also important to remember that eAG relates to plasma, not whole blood, so there will inevitably be some discrepancy with meter-based home blood glucose measurements. However, eAG could provide a more accessible estimate of control for patients and create the basis for more meaningful discussions about management.

cohort showed that for a mean blood glucose of 10 mmol/L based upon 7-point home blood glucose monitoring profiles over 24 hours, the HbA$_{1c}$ can range from 6% to 10%. A concept of rapid and slow glycators has been proposed to explain this phenomenon, but it is more likely to reflect variable red blood cell membrane transport of glucose. Recent research has shown a range of approximately 0.7–1.0 for this property between individuals and could explain HbA$_{1c}$ differences of 1.5–2.3% for any given mean blood glucose value. These observations question whether a single target HbA$_{1c}$ should be used and perhaps explains some of the often observed discrepancy between recorded home blood glucose tests and glycated haemoglobin concentrations.

The recommended frequency of testing of HbA$_{1c}$ is twice per year in stable patients and 4–6 times for those undergoing treatment changes.

Estimated average glucose (eAG)

Because many patients have difficulty relating HbA$_{1c}$ to their results of home blood glucose monitoring, glycated haemoglobin levels are now often reported together with an estimated average blood glucose (eAG). The initial equations were based upon the DCCT cohort but the more recently used conversion has come from the A1c-Derived Average Glucose (ADAG) Trial (Table 9.2) utilising frequent capillary blood glucose measurements and continuous subcutaneous blood glucose monitoring. The strongly positive correlation

Glucose variability

Attempts have been made to obtain an estimate of blood glucose variability based upon the ranges or standard deviations of the mean of profiles, or continuous subcutaneous monitoring. So far, these analyses using the DCCT and other data sets have not been shown to provide advantages over HbA$_{1c}$ alone.

IFCC standard

Most HbA$_{1c}$ assays have been standardised to that used in the DCCT as part of work carried out by the National Glycohaemoglobin Standardisation Programme (NGSP) in the USA. However, Sweden and Japan have each had their own standard. The IFCC has developed a new reference method that specifically measures only one molecular species of HbA$_{1c}$ and relates this to total haemoglobin. This method is expensive and laborious and can only be used to standardise local assays. It reports in units of mmol/mol and the absolute values will be quite different from the current familiar percentage. However, it has been decided internationally that there should be a gradual switch to the IFCC standard with its new units. An international consensus agreed the following.
- HbA$_{1c}$ results would be standardised worldwide to the new IFCC standard.
- The IFCC method is currently the only valid anchor that permits such standardisation.

Table 9.3 Guide to new values of HbA$_{1c}$ (IFCC) and DCCT (NGSP) standardised assay

DCCT %	New IFCC method (mmol/mol)
4.0	20
5.0	31
6.0	42
6.5	48
7.0	53
7.5	58
8.0	64
9.0	75
10.0	86

Conversion equation IFCC HbA$_{1c}$ (mmol/mol) = [DCCT HbA$_{1c}$ (%) − 2.15] × 10.929.

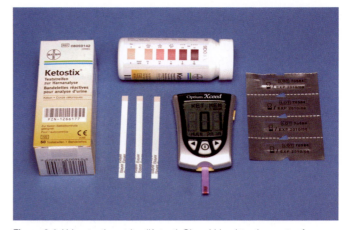

Figure 9.4 Urine testing strips (Ketostix®) and blood testing meter for ketones. NB urine tests detect acetoacetate; blood tests detect β hydroxybutyrate.

- HbA$_{1c}$ would be reported in both new and old units for the time being (probably until 2011) together with eAG.
- Glycaemic goals should be expressed in IFCC units, NGSP percent and eAG mmol/L or mg/dL.

Fructosamine

Serum fructosamine is a measure of glycated serum protein, mostly albumin, and is an indicator of glycaemic control over the preceding 2–3 weeks (the lifetime of albumin). Colorimetric assays for fructosamine, which are now adapted for automated analysers, give a normal reference range of 205–285 μmol/L. Fructosamine generally correlates well with HbA$_{1c}$, except when control has changed recently.

It has potential advantages over HbA$_{1c}$, particularly in situations such as haemoglobinopathies or pregnancy when the glycated haemoglobin is hard to interpret. However, standardisation is difficult: uraemia, lipaemia, hyperbilirubinaemia and vitamin C use can affect the assay, and there may be an effect of high or low circulating blood proteins.

Urine and blood ketone measurements

Ketones can be measured in urine using a colorimetric test or in capillary blood using an electrochemical sensor similar to those now used for glucose (Figure 9.4).

Acetoacetate and acetone are detected by the urine test, β hydroxybutyrate by the blood sensors. As the ratio of β hydroxybutyrate to acetoacetate is around 6:1 in human ketoacidosis, the blood sensor offers a convenient way to monitor diabetes control during intercurrent illness or in situations that may predispose to ketoacidosis, such as pregnancy, or where it can occur relatively quickly, such as in patients using continuous subcutaneous insulin infusion pump therapy. As yet there is little evidence on which to

CASE HISTORY

A 24-year-old white Europid man developed classic symptoms of type 1 diabetes and was commenced upon insulin as a basal–bolus regimen. His initial HbA$_{1c}$ was 9.7%. Six months later at regular review his home blood glucose monitoring showed excellent control with readings between 3.8 and 8.9 mmol/L (68–160 mg/dL) and he only reported occasional, mild, effort-related hypoglycaemia. However, his HbA$_{1c}$ value came back the next day at 8.3%. He was contacted at home and an increase in his insulin of 2 units per dose was recommended and a repeat HbA$_{1c}$ ordered for 6 weeks time. This was 8.1% and further insulin increase was instituted. Five days later he was admitted to hospital following a profound nocturnal hypoglycaemic episode during which he was found fitting.

Haemoglobin electrophoresis revealed the presence of HbS. The laboratory used an HbA$_{1c}$ assay that was sensitive to HbS, particularly at lower HbA$_{1c}$ concentrations. On direct questioning, it transpired that his parents were from the Mediterranean area.

Comment: Several learning points emerge. HbS can occur in non-African populations, so a family history in all people with diabetes is important. Secondly, it is important to know the limitations of the assays used by local laboratories. Lastly, in the presence of discrepancies between home monitoring and laboratory, do not always assume the patient's tests are incorrect.

form a consensus but blood ketone testing should be available in acute medical and obstetric assessment units as well as for inpatients with diabetes with intercurrent illnesses and perhaps as a means of monitoring response to treatment for diabetic ketoacidosis. Many units also provide their insulin pump users with blood ketone monitoring.

Continuous glucose monitoring systems

A major objective of diabetes research has been to provide continuous real-time monitoring of blood glucose so that insulin therapy can be matched to glycaemia. Ideally such a system would be linked to an insulin delivery device automatically, thus 'closing the loop'. In the last decade, huge strides have been made to achieve this goal but the current systems based upon capillary blood glucose monitoring technology using electron transfer do have their drawbacks.

Firstly, they are based upon measures of interstitial fluid, not blood glucose (Figure 9.5). This inevitably means that there is a delay or lag between detecting changes in blood glucose (mean delay 6.7 minutes, range 2–45 minutes). This lag can be affected by level of blood glucose, exercise, food intake and blood flow to the interstitial sampling site. Accuracy of the current devices tends to be less good at lower blood glucose levels. Secondly, such systems are by definition invasive as they require subcutaneous sensor insertion, usually on the abdominal wall. Thirdly, linkage to subcutaneous insulin infusion pumps introduces a further time lag in responsiveness (that of insulin absorption from the subcutaneous site). Finally, they need intermittent calibration with capillary blood glucose tests. The technology is also expensive and requires replacement every 5 days or so.

Clinical trials have, however, shown modest improvements of around 0.5% HbA$_{1c}$ at 6 months in young adults >25 years of age; children and adolescents in the same study showed no significant benefit. In a separate study, adults with an HbA$_{1c}$ <7% had a significant reduction in the time spent in biochemical hypoglycaemia when randomised to continuous glucose monitoring compared to intermittent capillary blood tests. However, there was no difference in

LANDMARK CLINICAL TRIAL

Koenig RJ, Peterson CM, Jones RL, Saudek C, Lehrman M, Cerami A. Correlation of glucose regulation and hemoglobin A1c in diabetes mellitus. N Engl J Med 1976; 295: 417–420.

Although abnormal haemoglobin electrophoresis had been described in diabetes since the 1950s, this was the first correlation between change in glycaemia and change in HbA$_{1c}$. Five patients with a fasting blood glucose ranging from 280 to 450 mg/dL (15.6–25.0 mmol/L) were hospitalized and their values corrected to 70–100 mg/dL (3.9–5.6 mmol/L). HbA$_{1c}$ was 6.8–12.1% initially, falling to 4.2–7.6% after glycaemic improvement. Later, much larger studies confirmed the linear relationship but the author's conclusion was spot on: 'Periodic monitoring of hemoglobin A$_{1c}$ levels provides a useful way of documenting the degree of control of glucose metabolism in diabetic patients …'.

KEY WEBSITES

- National Glycohemoglobin Support Program. Excellent information on HbA$_{1c}$, eAG and the new IFCC standards: www.ngsp.org
- National Institute for Health and Clinical Excellence (NICE). All UK guidelines available on this site (Type 1 Clinical Guidance CG15, Type 2 CG 66): www.nice.org.uk
- Diabetes UK. Guidance on monitoring: www.diabetes.org.uk
- American Diabetes Association. Standards of care published in *Diabetes Care* as a supplement each January: http://professional. diabetes.org/
- SIGN Guidelines: www.SIGN.ac.uk

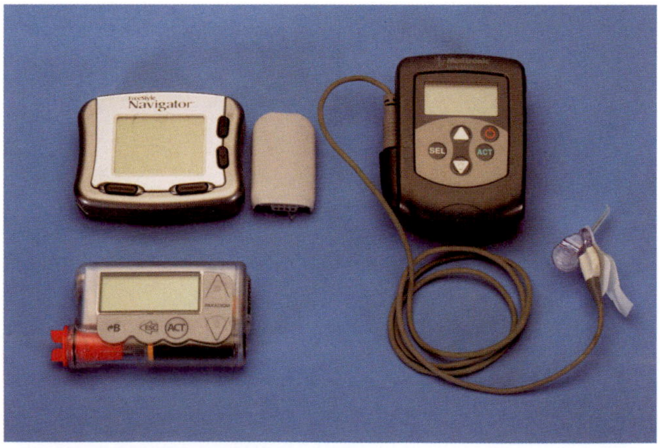

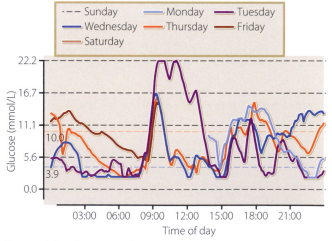

Figure 9.5 Examples of continuous interstitial glucose monitoring devices. Also shown is the Medtronic Veo subcutaneous insulin infusion pump with built in glucose sensor. Systems comprise a small subcutaneous sensor that communicates with a separate meter and screen or pump.

Figure 9.6 Sample print out of continuous glucose monitoring using Medtronic Gold sensor. Note the tendency for hypoglycaemia in early morning with large post prandial rise post breakfast and a smaller one post supper (1800 hours). Reduction in overnight insulin and increase in meal time boluses was initiated.

HbA$_{1c}$ in this study. These trials have used open loop algorithms and results were highly dependent upon patient motivation, training and education. Those who used the devices more consistently and made regular adjustments to their insulin dose obtained most benefit.

Closed loop devices and truly non-invasive glucose monitoring systems are under intense research and there are certain to be rapid developments in the near future. Meanwhile, the existing systems based upon interstitial glucose sensing probably have a role for patients struggling with glycaemic control (particularly those with unpredictable and severe hypoglycaemia), who are either on an insulin pump or multiple daily injections, and who are looked after by specialist teams who are well versed in the technology (Figure 9.6).

FURTHER READING

American Diabetes Association. Standards of medical care in diabetes – 2010. Diabetes Care 2010; 33(Suppl 1): S1–S100.

American Diabetes Association, European Association for the Study of Diabetes, International Federation of Clinical Chemistry and Laboratory Medicine, and International Diabetes Federation. Consensus statement on the world-wide standardisation of the HbA$_{1c}$ measurement. Diabetologia 2007; 50: 2042–2043.

Collier A, Ghosh D, Davidson DF, Kilpatrick ES. HbA$_{1c}$: 'the old order changeth'. Diabetic Med 2009; 26: 573–576.

DAFNE Study Group. Training in flexible, intensive insulin management to enable dietary freedom in people with type 1 diabetes : dose adjustment for normal eating (DAFNE) randomized controlled trial. BMJ 2002; 325:746–751.

Goldstein D, Little RR, Lorenz RA, et al. Tests of glycemia in diabetes. Diabetes Care 2004; 27: 1761–1773.

Khera PJ, Joiner CH, Carruthers A, et al. Evidence for individual heterogeneity in the glucose gradient across the human red blood cell membrane and its relationship to hemoglobin glycation. Diabetes 2008; 57: 2445–2452.

Nathan DM, Kunen J, Borg R, Zheng H, Schoenfeld D, Heine RJ, for the A1C Derived Average Glucose (ADAG) Study Group. Translating the A1C assay into estimated average glucose. Diabetes Care 2008; 31: 1473–1478.

National Collaborating Centre for Chronic Conditions. *Type 1 Diabetes in Adults*. London: Royal College of Physicians, 2006.

National Collaborating Centre for Chronic Conditions. *Type 2 Diabetes*. London: Royal College of Physicians, 2008.

Oliver NS, Toumazou C, Cass AEG, Johnston DG. Glucose sensors: a review of current and emerging technology. Diabetic Med 2009; 26: 197–210.

Reynolds TM, Smellie WSA, Twomey PJ. Glycated haemoglobin (HbA$_{1c}$) monitoring. BMJ 2006; 333: 586–588.

Welschen LMC, Bloemendal E, Nijpels G, et al. Self-monitoring of blood glucose in patients with type 2 diabetes mellitus who are not using insulin. Cochrane Database Syst Rev 2005; 3: CD005060.

Management of type 1 diabetes

KEY POINTS

- The objective of insulin treatment is to try and reproduce the physiological pattern of insulin production using subcutaneous injections. This usually entails multiple daily injections of short-, intermediate- or long-acting insulins, together with regular capillary blood glucose testing.
- There is no clear evidence-based superiority of the newer short- or long-acting insulin analogues in terms of glycaemic control.

- Continuous subcutaneous insulin infusion can improve glycaemia and reduce hypoglycaemia in patients struggling on conventional therapy.
- Islet transplantation (where it is available) could be considered for patients with severe disabling hypoglycaemia.

Modern management of type 1 diabetes comprises a package of measures including multiple daily injections for a more physiological insulin replacement; assessment of glycaemic control using blood glucose self-monitoring as well as clinic tests such as glycated haemoglobin (HbA$_{1c}$); insulin dosage adjustment according to diet and exercise; a healthy diet and carbohydrate counting; and intensive diabetes education. In the Diabetes Control and Complications Trial (DCCT) 1441 patients were randomised to either intensive treatment (including all the elements listed above plus regular contact with a named healthcare professional) or to conventional therapy with one or two injections of insulin a day. Significant improvements in HbA$_{1c}$ and a reduction in microvascular complications were seen in the intensively managed group. In practice, it is difficult to sustain the level of intensive healthcare professional support in the DCCT. In the UK the Diet Adjustment For Normal Eating (DAFNE) Programme comprising a 5-day intensive education programme has been shown to significantly reduce HbA$_{1c}$ at 6 and 12 months. Educational aspects of management such as these will be dealt with later (see Chapter 31).

Insulin replacement

The objective of insulin replacement is to mimic the insulin secretion pattern in the person without diabetes with mul-

tiple subcutaneous injections. In the person without diabetes, there is normally a rapid increase in plasma insulin after meals, triggered by glucose absorption into the bloodstream. This surge in insulin limits postprandial glycaemia by stimulating hepatic and peripheral glucose uptake. During fasting and between meals, insulin measurements drop to much lower levels (often called basal or steady state) which are sufficient to maintain blood glucose in the range 3.5–5.5 mmol/L. Even after a prolonged fast, it is possible to detect circulating insulin.

Basal insulin levels tend to be highest in the early morning, probably in response to the well-described surge in growth hormone and cortisol at that time of day (Figure 10.1). These counter-regulatory hormones tend to increase blood glucose and this has been termed the 'dawn phenomenon'.

For practical reasons, insulin is usually injected subcutaneously and regimens comprise short-acting (soluble, regular or analogue) insulin to simulate the normal mealtime surge, together with a longer acting insulin which is used to provide the background or basal concentration. This combination is called the 'basal-bolus' regimen or multiple daily injection (MDI) therapy (Figure 10.2).

Other routes of insulin administration such as intravenous infusion or intramuscular injection have not proven practical in the long term and despite intensive research, oral insulin preparations are not yet available.

Until the 1980s, insulin was extracted and purified from animal sources. Porcine and bovine insulins are still available

Handbook of Diabetes, 4th edition. By © Rudy Bilous & Richard Donnelly. Published 2010 by Blackwell Publishing Ltd.